Launching Your Career in Nutrition and Dietetics

SECOND EDITION

**Kyle Shadix, MS, RDN, CRC, FAND,
and Milton Stokes, PhD, MPH, RDN, FAND,
with Catherine Cioffi, RDN**

 press

Launching Your Career in Nutrition and Dietetics, Second Edition

ISBN 978-0-88091-992-0 (print)

ISBN 978-0-88091-993-7 (eBook)

ISBN 978-0-88091-987-6 (ePUB)

ISBN 978-0-88091-988-3 (PDF)

ISBN 978-0-88091-989-0 (Mobi)

Catalog Number 439017, 439017e

The views expressed in this publication are those of the authors and do not necessarily reflect policies and/or official positions of the Academy of Nutrition and Dietetics. Mention of product names in this publication does not constitute endorsement by the authors or the Academy of Nutrition and Dietetics. The Academy of Nutrition and Dietetics disclaims responsibility for the application of the information contained herein.

For more information on the Academy of Nutrition and Dietetics, visit www.eatright.org.

10 9 8 7 6 5 4 3 2 1

Library of Congress Cataloging-in-Publication Data

Names: Shadix, Kyle W., author. | Stokes, Milton, author. | Cioffi, Catherine, author. | Preceded by (work): Shadix, Kyle W. Launching your dietetics career. | Academy of Nutrition and Dietetics, issuing body.
Title: Launching your career in nutrition and dietetics: how to thrive in the classroom, the internship, and your first job / Kyle Shadix and Milton Stokes, with Catherine Cioffi.
Description: Second edition. | Chicago: Academy of Nutrition and Dietetics, 2016. | Preceded by: Launching your dietetics career / Kyle W. Shadix and D. Milton Stokes ; with Jenna A. Bell. c2011. | Includes bibliographical references and index.
Identifiers: LCCN 2016021761 (print) | LCCN 2016022095 (ebook) | ISBN 9780880919920 (print: alk. paper) | ISBN 9780880919937 (eBook)
Subjects: | MESH: Dietetics | Vocational Guidance
Classification: LCC RM218.5 (print) | LCC RM218.5 (ebook) | NLM WB 400 | DDC 613.2023—dc23
LC record available at https://lccn.loc.gov/2016021761

Contents

Acknowledgments

We are thrilled to have reached this exciting point—the second edition of *Launching Your Career in Nutrition and Dietetics*—and thank those who have joined and helped us on this endeavor!

We conceived the initial idea in 2002, sitting on a New York City bench outside Bubby's restaurant, thinking our entrepreneurial thoughts, imagining what our careers would look like if we could be anything in the world of nutrition and dietetics. Fast forward to today: Many interesting twists and turns presented themselves, including delightful characters and unexpected forks in the road, making the process feel slow and challenging at times, but also fast and fulfilling at others. And the journey isn't over!

Not only do we get the satisfaction of sharing our book idea in this handy guide, but we learned more than we ever imagined about personal and professional development, about persistence and patience, about writing and editing, and about how to enjoy and celebrate the outcome. I hope we never forget this meaningful experience.

We thank all of our monumental colleagues around the world who have helped us grow. They were doing all the wonderfully wild work in the real world of dietetics long before we thought about writing it all down, long before we wanted to encourage others in the profession to create new paradigms for work and careers. Many of those giants are featured in the "Movers and Shakers" chapter. And you know what they say about icebergs—we recognize that these are just an iceberg "tip" of worthy colleagues, and we wager you know someone who is just as formidable who inspired you, too. There's just so much positivity to go around!

We owe gratitude to Jenna Bell, PhD, RD, our friend, co-conspirator, and coauthor on the first edition of *Launching*. Kyle and I got the project off the ground; Jenna landed the plane to thunderous applause.

In preparing the second edition, we gained momentum from our intern, Liz Huseman. Then Catherine Cioffi wonderfully pulled it all together.

To the amazing publishing team at the Academy: Thank you for hanging in there with us through the duration.

And to our families: We appreciate all you've done to encourage us with this edition.

Last, to the reviewers who generously contributed their time and expertise, we thank you for your guidance and advice in shaping this new edition.

Brenda Eissenstat, MS, RD, LDN
Senior Instructor/Academic Adviser
Department of Nutritional Sciences
The Pennsylvania State University

Kathrin A. Eliot, PhD, RD, FAND
Assistant Professor and Director
Didactic Program in Dietetics
Saint Louis University

Janet Johnson, MS, RDN, LD
Senior Clinician
Iowa State University

Doris Piccinin, MS, RD, CDE
Clinical Nutritionist
Penn Medicine, Perelman Center for Advanced Medicine
Philadelphia, PA

Peggy Turner, MS, RD, LD, FAND
Assistant Professor
University of Oklahoma Health Sciences Center

About the Authors

Kyle Shadix

Chef Kyle Shadix is a certified research chef (CRC), registered dietitian (RDN), and fellow of the Academy of Nutrition and Dietetics (FAND). Chef Kyle supports new product development and innovation for PepsiCo R&D in Valhalla, NY. Previously, Chef Kyle was the founder of his own agency, Nutrition & Culinary Consultants, acquired in 2006 by WPP, the world's largest communication company.

Prior to that, Kyle's food and nutrition career has spanned from the drive-thru window at McDonald's in rural Georgia to New York City's acclaimed Bouley and the Gotham Bar & Grill. Kyle has also worked as an instructor at Columbia University, as an operations manager at Lehman Brothers, and at Memorial Sloan Kettering Cancer Center. In the past, Kyle has also served as the media spokesperson for companies including Dannon, the Mayo Clinic, Netflix, Celestial Seasonings, and the United States Tea Council. Kyle has served on the board of the American Institute of Wine and Food and has held numerous leadership positions for the Academy of Nutrition and Dietetics and the International Association of Culinary Professionals. Kyle has received various awards and recognition, such as the Academy's Recognized Young Dietitian of the Year award for New York state, the Emily Quinn Professional Achievement Award from the University of Georgia Alumni Association, and the Publix Visiting Practitioner at the University of Georgia's Department of Food and Nutrition.

As of this printing, Kyle is studying part time for his PhD in food science at Rutgers University, NJ; he expects to complete the program by 2019. He received his master's degree in foods and nutrition from New York University; bachelor's degree in consumer foods and food science from the University of Georgia, Athens; and culinary training at the Culinary Institute of America in Hyde Park, NY, and Le Cordon Bleu in Paris.

Milton Stokes

Milton Stokes is director of Global Health and Nutrition Outreach for Monsanto, where he engages with registered dietitian nutritionists and other health professionals on topics pertaining to food, agriculture, and nutrition. Before coming to Monsanto, Milton had a professorship and directed a dietetic internship at the University of Saint Joseph in West Hartford, CT. He also owned a private nutrition counseling practice with offices throughout Connecticut and is a former restauranteur.

Milton was a national media spokesperson for the Academy of Nutrition and Dietetics in the New York City media market and a freelance writer for consumer magazines covering food, nutrition, and health. Milton has authored several other books, including a *New York Times* best seller, *Flat Belly Diet! for Men* (2010).

Milton began his career in clinical nutrition in New York City with a food and nutrition management company. He has served in staff and management positions along the way as well as precepted dietetic interns and students from several colleges and programs. Milton's master's degree is in public health from Hunter College, and his clinical training was conducted at Yale New Haven Hospital affiliated with Yale University School of Medicine. Milton's doctoral degree from the University of Connecticut is in communication and marketing.

Visit him at www.miltonstokes.com, and follow him on Twitter @miltonstokes.

Catherine Cioffi

Catherine Cioffi is a registered dietitian nutritionist who began her nutrition career at Cornell University as an undergraduate nutritional sciences major. There she completed the accredited didactic program in dietetics, as well as the honors research program, and, upon graduating, was matched to the dietetic internship at Brigham and Women's Hospital in Boston, MA. Catherine became a registered dietitian nutritionist in the fall of 2013 and then spent two years working in the food industry at PepsiCo, Inc, in Westchester, NY, where her work in research and development focused on the translation of nutrition science for consumers and for product and business applications. Today, she is pursuing her PhD in nutrition and health sciences at Emory University in Atlanta, GA. She hopes to focus her research on childhood overweight and obesity, specifically weight management strategies and chronic disease prevention.

Foreword

This second edition of *Launching Your Career in Nutrition and Dietetics* by Kyle Shadix and Milton Stokes is a timely update, as the profession of nutrition and dietetics continues to expand and evolve, both in practice opportunities and consumer awareness.

In selecting a career in nutrition and dietetics, it's critical to first prepare yourself academically and for an internship and then to decide what area of nutrition and dietetics interests you most. Should you be a clinical dietitian or a public health nutritionist? Do you like being part of a dynamic foodservice environment? How about providing nutrition services to preschoolers or elderly clients? Maybe you would like to develop recipes and educational materials for a food or agriculture company, or maybe you would like to give supermarket tours. If social justice is your interest, then perhaps you want to help fight food insecurity. Does your curiosity about food intake patterns or nutrient functions steer you toward research? Is your dream job at a health and fitness facility, where you can provide group diabetes or diet and exercise classes? Maybe your proficiency in other languages is the key to consulting as a niche practitioner who translates nutrition education materials. These are just a few of the paths you may choose to follow! The registered dietitian nutritionists (referred to throught the book as RDNs) featured in Chapter 8, "Movers and Shakers," will give you a taste of some of the exciting opportunities within your reach.

A career in nutrition and dietetics offers many areas of practice, and you can choose to specialize or diversify. I chose to diversify and, over the course of my career, have worked as a clinical dietitian in medical, surgical, and obstetrics and gynecology units; in a clinic with expectant moms and babies; in an agency developing programs for grades K–12 and after-school programs; for companies developing recipes and educational materials; for a national health study training interviewers; for schools teaching nursing, foodservice, undergraduate, and graduate students, or workers at child-care centers; and for agencies developing culturally appropriate menus or messaging. In my current role as professor and chairperson of the Department of Nutrition and Dietetics at the University of North Florida, it has become obvious to me that students need straightforward guidance from experienced dietetics practitioners. This helps students effectively plan their studies, be prepared to apply for and succeed in an internship, and gain the knowledge and skills they need for successful completion of the RDN exam and entry into the profession. Moreover, while serving as President of the Academy of Nutrition and Dietetics (then the American Dietetic Association), I met hundreds of practitioners in a wide range of work settings. I also saw that when students know the many career options available to them, they become even more excited about their chosen career!

This latest edition of *Launching Your Career in Nutrition and Dietetics* provides a template for your studies as well as the selection and application process for a supervised practice experience (dietetic internship). Throughout the book, you will find tips for gaining valuable extracurricular experiences to help you develop a competitive dietetic internship application and launch your career. Above all, this book encourages you to seek additional experiences—ask your professors, shadow practitioners, attend professional meetings—to learn more about what interests you. But don't stop there: Investigate areas that you *think* might not interest you—and you may be surprised with the results.

Many thanks to Milton and Kyle for writing, and now updating, this essential guide. I have long admired their enthusiasm for and dedication to the profession. Even more admirable is their commitment to mentoring and helping others "learn the ropes." Their advice can help you successfully navigate your studies, the internship application, and passing the registration exam and can give you a comprehensive idea of the many opportunities the profession has to offer.

Best wishes for success and a long and fulfilling career in nutrition and dietetics.

Judith Rodriguez, PhD, RD
Professor and Chair, Department of Nutrition and Dietetics, University of North Florida
Past President, Academy of Nutrition and Dietetics (2010–2011)

Introduction

Greetings! We are pleased to be your tour guides as you navigate the path from dietetics student to dietetics intern and ultimately to practicing dietitian. We created this book because we wish we'd had an instruction manual like this when we were learning the ropes. Now that we're practicing and thriving in this exciting profession, we'd like to share our insights and experiences so your career journey can be a bit smoother.

In its second edition, this book provides the latest information you'll need for entering and advancing in the field of nutrition and dietetics. While some of the information you'll find in this book can be found online (and we've provided many links to guide you), we think you'll agree that having it all in one place can be a significant time-saver. Along with the practical information, we've included candid advice and inspiration from several of our esteemed colleagues, including a chapter devoted to tips and advice for success from some "movers and shakers" in the field.

Our goal is to help you stay energized, focused, and productive on your journey to becoming a registered dietitian nutritionist. We hope you love the end result—being a dietitian—as much as we do!

CHAPTER 1

Welcome to Nutrition and Dietetics!

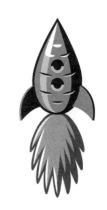

THOUGHT QUESTIONS

- Why are you interested in the field of food and nutrition? Was it one experience, personal or professional, or a combination of many reasons?

- Have you ever met a registered dietitian nutritionist? If so, what professional sector does he or she work in, and in what role? If not, search the Internet for a current registered dietitian nutritionist and describe his or her line of work.

- What would you like to do as a registered dietitian

C ONGRATULATIONS! BY OPENING THIS BOOK, YOU'VE taken a smart path to learning about a career in nutrition and dietetics—a dynamic profession projected to grow 16% from 2014 to 2024, according to the Bureau of Labor Statistics. With increasing awareness of the role of healthful diet and lifestyle choices in preventing chronic diseases and improving quality of life, there have never been more diverse opportunities in the field of nutrition. As of 2014, almost 67,000 registered dietitian nutritionists (RDNs) were actively working as food and nutrition experts in a variety of general areas: clinical and health care, community and public health, academia, research, food service, food and nutrition management, retail, private practice, food industry, media and communication, and many more.[1]

A Spectrum of Career Choices

If you have a passion for food and health, pursuing a career in nutrition and dietetics may be a perfect option for you. As you will see from the various work environments and job functions described next, no single personality type is required for success in this field. The dietetics profession can suit a range of interests, preferences, and styles. Yet, the work of RDNs (sometimes referred to as RDs) is unified by an emphasis on science- and evidence-based practice and effective communication skills, as well as teamwork, critical thinking, and patient- and/or client-centered service.

Clinical and Health Care Dietitians

A large percentage of RDNs work in a clinical or health care setting. According to the Bureau of Labor Statistics, 30% of dietitians are employed at hospitals, followed by 10% at nursing and long-term care facilities and 8% at outpatient clinics.[1] Clinical dietitians assess nutritional needs; provide nutrition diagnoses; develop and implement nutrition plans to address needs; and then monitor, evaluate, and adjust plans along the way as needed. This systematic approach, called the Nutrition Care Process (NCP), is the foundation of medical nutrition therapy.

Clinical RDNs work with doctors, nurses, speech pathologists, and other health care professionals as part of a coordinated team. In addition to ensuring that patients' nutritional needs are met, they also provide nutrition education based on a patient's specific condition. Areas of specialization include cardiovascular health, weight management, kidney (renal) disease, diabetes, oncology, burns or trauma, pediatrics, and critical care.

Primary care settings have also grown as an opportunity for RDNs to work on teams with other health practitioners. This has stemmed from a new model of health care called patient-centered medical care—a comprehensive approach to primary care that strives to be "patient-centered, team-based, coordinated, accessible, and focused on quality and safety."[2] It also endorses prevention and wellness services, including access to nutritional counseling.

Community and Public Health Dietitians

RDNs work in community and public health settings where they assume a range of roles that all function to promote healthful eating habits and improve quality of life in public health. They may work in food banks, schools, corrections facilities, advocacy organizations, community clinics, home health agencies, and other food and health organizations. Public health–related opportunities are available at government assistance programs, such as the Special Supplemental Nutrition Program for Women, Infants, and Children (WIC), Supplemental Nutrition Assistance Program (SNAP) education initiatives, or at cooperative extension programs managed by land-grant colleges and universities in surrounding communities.[3] Much as clinical dietitians do, community dietitians follow the NCP by assessing the nutritional needs of their audience and developing appropriate nutrition care plans and interventions. This may comprise nutrition education to individuals and groups, in-home counseling on grocery shopping and food preparation to low-income or other at-risk groups, collaboration with community farmers markets to promote access to fresh produce, service as a subject matter expert to advise an organization's nutrition policies or advocacy efforts, and many others!

Food and Nutrition Management Dietitians

Foodservice management dietitians are the gatekeepers of food safety, kitchen safety, menu development, budgeting, and planning for small- to large-scale hospitals, companies, and corporate sites. As managers, they may hire, train, and direct other RDNs and foodservice workers. Especially in recent years, interest in the nutrition quality of foods has led to larger efforts to revolutionize food service, from developing more healthful, tasty choices by collaborating with chefs to providing education through labeling and on-site presentations or demonstrations to inform food choices. More upscale foodservice establishments, such as restaurant groups and wineries, hire dietitians to act as subject matter experts in nutrition and health. Federal legislation in the form of the Healthy, Hunger-Free Kids Act of 2010 has emphasized improving the nutrition quality of the National School Lunch and Breakfast Programs, creating a need for foodservice dietitians in school dining settings.[4]

Dietitians also hold management positions in clinical nutrition settings, such as in hospitals or other health care settings. For example, a clinical nutrition manager plans, coordinates, and manages the work operations of the clinical nutrition staff. This position also works closely with foodservice managers to ensure that nutrition needs of patients or residents are met. A director or manager in clinical nutrition settings is responsible for ensuring the provision of optimal, cost-effective patient nutrition care through recruiting, hiring, and managing staff and working closely with hospital or facility leadership.

Academic, University, and Research Dietitians

Academic and research dietitians typically work in universities or medical centers by directing or conducting research to answer critical food- and nutrition-related questions and to evaluate current nutrition recommendations and guidelines. This might be clinical lab research, often in conjunction with a hospital or medical center, as well as other types of research, such as community intervention studies, program evaluations, epidemiology and observational research, and others. Academic dietitians may also be involved in nutrition education, curriculum development, and teaching as faculty of a college or university nutrition department. There are also faculty opportunities in other areas, such as in culinary schools and in medical or nursing schools—fields that are increasingly collaborating with dietetics professionals and incorporating health and nutrition education into their professional training.

Retail and Food Industry Dietitians

RDNs are sought in food and health retail settings, such as supermarkets, grocery stores, and drug stores. Retail dietitians work with a variety of audiences, from educating customers about healthful eating and providing personalized nutrition advice, to implementing wellness programs for employees, to advocating for nutrition among senior executives. The Retail Dietitians Business Alliance (RDBA)—the professional organization for retail RDNs—proposes that the retail dietitian is "uniquely positioned to profoundly impact public health while at the same time supporting the business of food retail."[5]

Other jobs in the food industry and business can be found at food and beverage, pharmaceutical, and supplement manufacturing companies or in food commodity and agricultural organizations that represent food groups or food categories. These positions emphasize communication and outreach, public relations, nutrition labeling and regulatory expertise, public policy, commercial writing, advertising, and marketing. There are also opportunities in research and development, where RDNs collaborate with food scientists to create more healthful product offerings.

Consultant and Private Practice Dietitians

Consultant dietitians have limitless opportunities, typically working under a consultancy agreement or owning their own company. As entrepreneurs, some work under contract with hospitals, doctors' offices, or long-term-care centers. Some run their own private practices, where they conduct nutrition screenings and assessments and then provide nutrition counseling to their private clients to treat and prevent disease or poor health. Others may be consultants for worksite wellness programs, professional or collegiate sports teams, and supermarkets. Some serve as media spokespersons for food and beverage companies, trade associations, or other health- and wellness-related organizations; others are nutrition writers for blogs, magazines, books, and other publications. Dietitians are increasingly business and technology savvy, developing and selling mobile apps and other online or social media resources as well as print products. The possibilities are endless. Because these dietitians are independent contractors or business owners, work ethic, time management, business knowledge, and networking are especially important factors for success in this area of practice.

RDN, RD, OR NUTRITIONIST: WHAT'S THE DIFFERENCE?

All registered dietitians are nutritionists, but not all nutritionists are registered dietitians.

The registered dietitian nutritionist (RDN) or registered dietitian (RD) credentials are interchangeable, legally protected titles. Only dietetics professionals who have completed the requirements of the Commission on Dietetic Registration can call themselves an RDN or RD—credentials that represent competence to provide services to patients and clients.*

The title of nutritionist, however, is unregulated. Do a quick search for "nutritionist" online to get an idea of the number of folks who do not bring the same assurances of accredited education and practice expertise as those qualified as RDNs or RDs.

*The RDN credential was offered as an option, beginning in 2013, to RDs who want to emphasize the nutrition aspect of their credential to the public and to other health practitioners. Although dietitians may choose the credential (RDN or RD) they wish to use in their practice, RDN will be used throughout this book.

Wellness and Sports Nutrition Dietitians

This growing area of practice focuses on education and counseling for the connections between food, fitness, and health. Wellness dietitians may work as consultants or may be employed by corporations, insurance companies, or health club facilities where they focus on ways to promote proactive lifestyles through both physical activity and healthful eating, in turn helping to prevent (or treat) chronic diseases, assist with weight management, improve quality of life and longevity, and reduce health care costs. Some dietitians choose to obtain a specialty certification in personal fitness or as a health coach to expand their skills in educating and supporting clients in achieving health goals. Sports dietitians provide "nutrition counseling and education to enhance the performance of competitive and recreational athletes," according to the Sports, Cardiovascular, and Wellness Nutrition (SCAN) dietetic practice group—a specialty group within the Academy of Nutrition and Dietetics. See Chapter 6 for more about dietetic practice groups.

What Qualifies a Registered Dietitian Nutritionist?

The eligibility criteria to be an RDN are established by the Commission on Dietetic Registration (CDR). Although requirements may change, currently, all RDN must have accomplished the following:

- completed a minimum of a bachelor's degree at a US regionally accredited university or college or foreign equivalent, as well as the required course work approved by the Accreditation Council for Education in Nutrition and Dietetics (ACEND), referred to as didactic programs in dietetics (DPDs) or coordinated programs (CPs) in dietetics;
- completed an ACEND-accredited supervised practice program through an accredited program at a health care facility, community agency, or foodservice corporation or combined with undergraduate or graduate studies (The supervised practice program typically runs 6 to 12 months in length.);
- passed a national examination administered by CDR; and
- completed continuing professional educational requirements to maintain the RDN/RD credential.[11]

Be aware that by 2024, the eligibility requirements for entry-level dietitians will be elevated from completion of a bachelor's degree to completion of a graduate degree. Read more about this upcoming change in Chapter 2. For more information about current and future requirements, visit the CDR website (www.cdrnet.org/entry-level).

What Is Supervised Practice?

The supervised practice requirements are most commonly fulfilled through an ACEND-accredited dietetic internship (DI), during which interns complete at least 1,200 hours of supervised practice. The DI takes place after the baccalaureate degree (or graduate degree) and DPD course work have been completed.

The supervised practice requirements can also be completed as part of a CP—another ACEND-accredited academic program offered at certain US colleges and universities. A CP integrates didactic

EMERGING OPPORTUNITIES: TELENUTRITION AND NUTRITION INFORMATICS

Telehealth is a type of virtual health care, defined as "the use of electronic information and telecommunication technologies to support long-distance health care, patient, and professional health-related education, public health, and health administration."[6] More specifically, the Academy of Nutrition and Dietetics defines telenutrition as the interactive use of digital technologies, such as videoconferencing, e-mail, and other electronic resources, by RDNs to implement the NCP with patients or clients at remote locations.[7] An evidence analysis review completed in 2012 by the Academy concluded that, "consistent evidence reports that telenutrition interventions and counseling provided by a registered dietitian resulted in significant improvements in weight, [body mass index], and other health outcomes," although the body of research in this area was still limited at the time.[8] As technology continues to evolve, state licensure boards and the Academy are working to resolve issues such as insurance coverage and licensure requirements. Here are a few things to know for now:

- The Centers for Medicare & Medicaid Services (CMS) recognizes and covers certain telehealth services, including medical nutrition therapy (MNT) and diabetes self-management training (DSMT), under Medicare Part B.

course work and the minimum 1,200 hours of supervised practice within one degree program, typically a baccalaureate degree. Certain DI or CP programs also result in a graduate degree, though these take longer to complete.

To meet the growing volume of applicants in recent years, starting in 2011, dietetics programs began offering an alternative for supervised practice called individualized supervised practice pathways (ISPPs).[12] Intended for self-directed students who completed the DPD course work but were not matched to a DI, ISPPs offer another option for students to gain the skills required to become an RDN. Certain ISPPs, but not all, can also be completed by qualified individuals with doctoral degrees who have not obtained a DPD verification statement but who can demonstrate they have achieved

- When providing telehealth services, RDNs must comply with regulations in the state where the client or patient resides. Multiple state licenses may be necessary if providing services in different states.

- To determine if you should add telenutrition to your practice, the Academy's Scope of Practice Decision Tool is available for purchase online.[9] This interactive tool can help RDNs determine whether a particular activity is within their scope of practice by critically evaluating their knowledge, skills, and competence.

Nutrition informatics is another emerging area, defined as "the effective retrieval, organization, storage, and optimum use of information, data, and knowledge for food and nutrition related problem solving and decision making. Informatics is supported by the use of information standards, processes and technology."[7] Put in simple terms, it is the intersection of nutrition, information, and technology. Current use of informatics in health care includes electronic medical records, outcomes-based research, and knowledge acquisition.[10] To be successful in the current and future health environment, dietitians must keep up with technological advances and applications relating to finding, evaluating, and sharing accurate food and nutrition information.

WHO'S WHO IN DIETETICS? IMPORTANT ORGANIZATIONS AND AGENCIES

Academy of Nutrition and Dietetics (Academy)

Founded in 1917, the Academy of Nutrition and Dietetics, is the largest professional organization for registered dietitian nutritionists (RDNs); nutrition and dietetic technicians, registered (NDTRs); students; and other related professionals.

The Academy is committed to improving the nation's health and advancing the profession of dietetics through advocacy, research, and education. To benefit members, the Academy offers various resources, services, and events to assist in developing skills, advancing knowledge, and achieving professional career goals.

Website: www.eatrightpro.org

Commission on Dietetic Registration (CDR)

CDR is the credentialing authority for RDNs as well as other legally protected credentials. It operates as a separate entity from the Academy, with an 11-member board that includes RDNs, NDTRs, and a public representative.

The CDR's mission is to protect the public by awarding credentials only to qualified candidates who have completed the necessary requirements and who have passed the registration examination. Beyond overseeing the credentialing processes, the CDR also supports lifelong learning and career advancement.

Website: www.cdrnet.org

Accreditation Council for Education in Nutrition and Dietetics (ACEND)

ACEND is an Academy-affiliated accrediting agency for all nutrition and dietetics education programs that prepare students for careers as RDNs and NDTRs.

In this role, ACEND establishes and enforces the eligibility requirements and accreditation standards for academic programs in nutrition and dietetics to ensure they are high quality, valued, and respected. ACEND also continually evaluates and revises accreditation standards based on trends in dietetics practice and to ensure fair accreditation decisions.

Website: www.eatrightacend.org

the knowledge requirements of a DPD through education or work experience.

More information about the different pathways to becoming an RDN will be covered in the next chapters. After supervised practice, all RDN candidates must pass CDR's registration exam to be granted the legally protected RDN credential. Many states also require licensure or offer certification in the interest of the public to protect against unqualified practitioners. When the time comes, it's wise to check with your state for details.

What Is a Nutrition and Dietetics Technician, Registered?

Although this book will focus on what it takes to become an RDN, you should know that there is another legally protected and dietetics-related credential offered by CDR: the nutrition and dietetics technician, registered (NDTR), also referred to as dietetic technician, registered (DTR). NDTRs are trained at the technical level of nutrition and dietetics practice and are capable of providing safe and quality nutrition services. They must complete an ACEND-accredited program that offers the academic course work, 450 hours of supervised practice experience (versus the 1,200 hours required for RDNs), and at least an associate's degree before being eligible to take the Registration Examination for Dietetic Technicians. Individuals who complete a DPD may also be eligible to sit for the NDTR exam. The NDTR can work in many of the same settings as the RDN, including hospitals, schools, community nutrition programs, and food companies but cannot perform all of the same duties. In some employment settings, NDTRs must work under the supervision of an RDN, especially if providing direct patient care to nutritionally at-risk populations. But in other settings, they may work independently, for example, providing nutrition education to healthy populations. For more information about becoming an NDTR, visit the CDR and ACEND websites (www.cdrnet.org and www.eatrightacend.org, respectively).

A Closer Look

RDNs Who Love Food: A Three-Step Process

By Jonathan Deutsch, PhD

For the past decade, I have been teaching food and cooking classes to nutrition students in DPD programs. That may sound like a fun and easy job. After all, such students are planning to devote their careers to food—won't they love to learn about food and cooking? For a surprising number of students, the answer is *no*, at least not at first. While nutrition students may be passionate about aspects of nutrition and nutrition science—encouraging healthful lifestyles in our communities, helping individuals change dietary behavior, and understanding the medical applications of diet—far fewer, it seems, actually want to become RDNs because they love to cook and eat and want to encourage others to do the same!

But is it necessary to love food and cooking to be an RDN? To illustrate how deeply held our individual and collective relationships with food are, I typically ask my students to write about a food that they would never eat and why they would never eat it. You, the reader, might want to try this as well. Class responses range from vegetables and fruits like okra, squash, and durian (a [foul]-smelling fruit), to meats and meat products like pork, tripe, or chitterlings, to cuisines and preparations like Korean food, sushi, or roasted grasshoppers. Next we discuss what factors contribute to the class's strong feelings against these foods. Some answers are as follows:

- "strange" texture
- religious prohibitions
- family memories
- personal negative experiences
- a "funny feeling"
- perceived healthfulness
- cultural preferences
- taste and personal preferences
- aroma
- connection to the living food system
- perceived food safety
- unfamiliarity

How do these factors compare to your reasons?

The need for food is not our only primary biological drive, but it is a central and potent channel of communication that carries a rich web of intentions, meanings, and larger forces influencing the way we eat. Culture, religion, psychology, nutrition, agriculture, economics, marketing, history, and politics all meet around the dinner table to shape how we eat. How we procure, prepare, and serve food is often powerfully negotiated in ways that address larger issues of gender, class, labor, and cultural identities.

Recognizing the importance, power, and prominence of food in our lives is the first step to becoming an RDN with an understanding of and relationship with food. I encourage aspiring RDNs to work through a three-step progression in their relationship with food: understanding, respect, and love.

1. **Understanding** is the bare minimum required in an RDN's relationship with food. It is the level required by the practice experience and examination to become an RDN. RDNs must be able to understand the physical and chemical properties of foods themselves; what happens to these properties during cooking, holding, and service; what to look for in purchasing foods; how to prepare foods in a safe and sanitary way; and how to follow procedures such as recipes, formulas, and foodservice systems and how to train others to do so as well.

Why Understanding? Such an understanding allows RDNs to work safely in hospital and foodservice settings. In a counseling capacity, it allows them to confidently recommend foods and preparations for a client's safe and healthful diet. In food service, it allows them to help chefs and foodservice workers select the best possible ingredients and prepare them in a way that best preserves the flavor, nutritional properties, and texture of the foods.

2. **Respect** for food, cooking, and eating makes a good RDN better. Having respect for food provokes the RDN to explain the *why* question with clients, foodservice workers, and communities to help them better understand and change dietary behavior. Any nutrition student who has taken an introductory foods course knows, for example, that fat plays an important role in "mouth feel," satiety, cooking properties, and flavor. An RDN who understands this may prescribe a reduced-fat diet for a specific client or setting, whereas one who respects these properties

CONTINUED ›

A CLOSER LOOK (CONTINUED) ┈┈┈┈┈┈┈┈┈┈┈┈┈┈┈┈┈┈┈┈┈┈┈┈┈┈┈┈┈┈┈┈

will be able to analyze the functions that fat is currently serving and at the same time recommend dietary change in a way that is appealing and fits with a client's personal preferences, lifestyle, and customs.

Why Respect? In our increasingly diverse world, nutrition wisdom needs to be contextualized for each client and setting. "Eat more fiber" is a less effective recommendation than providing some appealing, easy, cost-effective, flavorful, and culturally specific high-fiber recipes. Understanding not only what people are eating but also the nutritional, social, cultural, economic, and political *why* helps RDNs have a bigger impact. By respecting the food and food habits of an individual or community, RDNs can put their nutrition knowledge into action in a way that appeals to clients. Appealing recommendations, programs, and menus are more successful!

3. **Love** for food, cooking, and eating make the consummate RDN. An RDN's passion for a perfectly grilled steak, a vine-ripened tomato eaten whole in the garden, or the pleasure of bok choy steamed with ginger and garlic can inspire a client or class to share in that passion. Such passion can enable positive nutrition advice—instead of simply asking clients to eat less in general or less or more of specific nutrients, RDNs can encourage people to eat better by inspiring them and getting them excited about healthful eating.

Why Love? Loving food allows RDNs to innovate not only in programming but also in menus and culinary applications of food. An RDN who loves food, cooking, and eating can be "holistic" by first understanding the foods and their properties throughout the cycle; respecting these properties and their cultural, social, and personal values; and loving the foods, the pleasures of the table, and the sensual properties of food shopping, cooking, eating, and serving. In the same way that a passionate teacher can inspire a love of learning in his or her students, an RDN who is passionate about food can inspire a healthful and respectful relationship with food in his or her clients and communities.

Jonathan Deutsch is a professor of culinary arts and food science at Drexel University in Philadelphia.

References

1. Bureau of Labor Statistics, US Department of Labor. Occupational outlook handbook, 2016–17 edition, dietitians and nutritionists. http://www.bls.gov/ooh/healthcare/dietitians-and-nutritionists.htm. Published December 17, 2015. Accessed January 10, 2016.

2. Scholle SH, Torda P, Peikes D, Han E, Genevro J. *Engaging Patients and Families in the Medical Home.* AHRQ Publication No. 10-0083-EF. Rockville, MD: Agency for Healthcare Research and Quality. https://www.pcmh.ahrq.gov/page/engaging-patients-and-families-medical-home. Published June 2010. Accessed January 10, 2016.

3. US Department of Agriculture, National Institute of Food and Agriculture. Extension. http://nifa.usda.gov/Extension/. Accessed January 10, 2016.

4. US Department of Agriculture, Food and Nutrition Service. School meals: Healthy Hunger-Free Kids Act. http://www.fns.usda.gov/school-meals/healthy-hunger-free-kids-act. Published March 3, 2014. Accessed January 10, 2016.

5. Retail Dietitians Business Alliance (RDBA). About RDBA. http://www.retaildietitians.com/about/. Copyright 2013. Accessed January 10, 2016.

6. Academy of Nutrition and Dietetics. Telehealth. http://www.eatrightpro.org/resource/practice/getting-paid/emerging-health-care-delivery-and-payment/telehealth. Accessed January 10, 2016.

7. Academy of Nutrition and Dietetics, Quality Management Committee. Definition of terms list. http://www.eatrightpro.org/~/media/eatrightpro%20files/practice/scope%20standards%20of%20practice/definition%20of%20terms%20list.ashx. Updated January 2016. Accessed January 10, 2016.

8. Academy of Nutrition and Dietetics Evidence Analysis Library. TN: Telenutrition interventions by registered dietitians (2012). http://www.andeal.org/topic.cfm?menu=4706&cat=4907. Accessed January 10, 2016.

9. Academy of Nutrition and Dietetics. Scope of Practice Decision Tool. http://www.eatrightstore.org/product/051ECA8D-389E-478D-BD29-D259DB3AB295. Accessed January 10, 2016.

10. Charney P. Practice paper of the Academy of Nutrition and Dietetics abstract: nutrition informatics. *J Acad Nutr Diet.* 2012;112(11):1859. doi:10.1016/j.jand.2012.09.002.

11. Commission on Dietetics Registration. Registration eligibility requirements for dietitians. https://www.cdrnet.org/certifications /registration-eligibility-requirements-for-dietitians. Accessed January 10, 2016.

12. Accreditation Council for Education in Nutrition and Dietetics. Individualized supervised practice pathways (ISPPs). http://www .eatrightacend.org/ACEND/content.aspx?id=6442485529. Accessed January 10, 2016.

CHAPTER 2

Hitting the Books: Academic Requirements

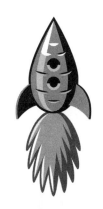

THOUGHT QUESTIONS

- Based on where you are in your career, do you understand the educational requirements necessary to become a registered dietitian nutritionist? Describe your options.

- Are there specific accredited undergraduate didactic programs in dietetics or coordinated programs in dietetics that you are already considering? Describe the course curriculum and other requirements, special emphases, or activities involved in these programs.

- Brainstorm three to five "outside" activities that you might consider to get involved in, such as volunteering, nonpaid or paid internship experience, independent study, and so forth.

O NCE YOU'VE MADE THE CHOICE TO FOLLOW YOUR PASSION
for nutrition, you'll want to select an academic program that's
right for you. Rest assured: Registered dietitian nutritionists
(RDNs) come from many backgrounds and life stages, and there are
a variety of pathways to choose from. This chapter will provide an
overview of the academic requirements you need to complete prior to
starting supervised practice. It will answer the following important
questions:

- If I'm a high school or college student, what type of degree
  should I pursue?
- If I'm changing careers, where should I start, and what course
  work do I need to complete?
- What extracurricular activities should I get involved in to be
  a qualified candidate for the supervised practice component?

Overview of Nutrition and Dietetics Education

The Accreditation Council for Education in Nutrition and Dietetics
(ACEND), an affiliate of the Academy of Nutrition and Dietetics, is
the accrediting agency for nutrition and dietetics education. The
purpose of accreditation is to ensure that dietetics programs meet
the standards for providing knowledge, skills, and other competencies that students need to become an entry-level RDN. As we
introduced in Chapter 1, to be qualified to take the registration examination, you must

- hold at least a bachelor's degree,
- have completed course work from either ACEND-accredited
  didactic programs in dietetics (DPDs) or coordinated programs (CPs) in dietetics, and
- have completed an ACEND-accredited supervised practice
  program offering at least 1,200 hours of supervised practice
  experience.[1]

It is important to note that there are multiple programs and
sequences for completing these requirements. Figure 2.1 shows the
two most common pathways. In the future, these standards and

requirements may change. For up-to-date information, visit the ACEND website (www.eatrightacend.org)—a section of the Academy of Nutrition and Dietetics website with specific pages and information designed for students.[1] This will be an important resource for your pursuit of a career in nutrition and dietetics.

FIGURE 2.1.
Accredited pathways for becoming a registered dietitian nutritionist

Pathway 1: Didactic Program Followed by Dietetic Internship

Didactic Program in Dietetics (DPD):
Required course work at bachelor's or graduate level, completed before supervised practice

Dietetic Internship (DI):
At least 1,200 supervised practice hours post-bachelor's degree, completed after the DPD course work

Coordinated Program in Dietetics (CP):
Combines required course work and supervised practice hours in one integrated program; students also obtain bachelor's or graduate-level degree

An ACEND-accredited DPD provides the academic classes you must complete before applying to an ACEND-accredited supervised practice program, also called the dietetic internship (DI). To gain accreditation, the program's course work must cover the required knowledge areas in food, nutrition, foodservice management, clinical care, community care, health care systems, and other health sciences. Although course titles may vary from one university to another, as shown in Figure 2.2, the overall curriculum and experiences will be similar.

DID YOU KNOW? The word *didactic* comes from the Greek *didaktikos*, which means literally "to teach." The didactic program in dietetics provides the academic or classroom learning necessary to teach future RDNs the knowledge they need to enter into a supervised practice, where they apply this knowledge to practice.

Fortunately for aspiring RDNs, there are more than 200 accredited DPDs in the United States, most of which are targeted to incoming undergraduate students who have not yet completed a bachelor's degree. A listing of all ACEND-accredited DPDs can be found on ACEND's website.[2] There are also graduate-level programs for individuals who are changing careers or already have a bachelor's degree.

In this first pathway, once the DPD is completed, you may then apply for DIs to complete the supervised practice requirements. The DI and the process of applying to DIs will be covered in depth in Chapters 3 and 4.

Pathway 2: Coordinated Programs Integrating Didactic Knowledge and Supervised Practice

An ACEND-accredited CP integrates the didactic course work and the required 1,200 hours of supervised practice into one program. CPs are an efficient option and are ideal for students who know early on that they want to become an RDN. For an undergraduate program, students typically apply to enroll in a CP during their freshman or sophomore year. If accepted, the timing and sequence of course work and supervised practice hours will vary depending on the program, but both are completed prior to graduation with a bachelor's degree. For a graduate-level program, prospective students may apply directly into the CP and then begin the requirements right away. Where possible, graduate schools will transfer course credits from prior institutions that qualify toward the degree or the ACEND competencies. It is best to work with the CP director for personalized academic planning.

FIGURE 2.2.
Sample didactic programs in dietetics course listings

Sample DPD Courses at University A		Sample DPD Courses at University B	
COURSE	CREDITS	COURSE	CREDITS
Biostatistics	3	Introduction to Modern Chemistry	5
Chemistry of Food	3	Principles of Organic Chemistry	5
Food Policy and Food Safety	3	Food Microbiology and Sanitation	3
Food Policy and Food Safety Lab	2	Nutritional Biochemistry	3
Protein and Carbohydrate	4	Principles of Human Anatomy and Physiology	3
Lipid Metabolism	4	Nutrition and Health	3
Vitamin and Mineral Nutrition	4	Diet Assessment and Planning	3
Evaluation of Nutrition Status	3	Nutrition and the Life Cycle	3
Community Nutrition	3	Clinical Nutrition Assessment and Intervention	3
Nutrition Education Principles	3	Community Nutrition	3
Nutrition and Chronic Disease	4	Introduction to Food Science	3
Medical Nutrition Therapy I	2	Food Management Theory	3
Nutrition in Acute Care	4	Food Production and Management	3
Medical Nutrition Therapy II	2	Food Science and Technology	3
Management of Nutrition Services	4		

RESEARCHING PROGRAMS: THE BASICS

The Academy of Nutrition and Dietetics offers an online resource with information about ACEND-accredited DPDs and CPs, where you can sort programs by state and certain features, such as whether they offer distance education or course credit transfer agreements or whether they result in a graduate degree. Below is a digital screenshot of ACEND's search tool for didactic programs in dietetics (DPDs).[2] We highly recommend visiting this resource—with so many programs to choose from, it is helpful having a tool to view the options!

STAY INFORMED

Didactic Programs in Dietetics

Listed below are the Didactic Programs in Dietetics (DPD). After each program's address is the status granted by the Accreditation Council for Education in Nutrition and Dietetics (ACEND) and the date of the next program review. The Accreditation status definitions are as follows:

- Candidacy for Accreditation—program not previously accredited that has had one site visit and is being implemented according to the ACEND Accreditation Standards.
- Accredited—program that has had at least one site visit and is in compliance with the Accreditation Standards.
- Probationary Accreditation—program fails to comply with the Accreditation Standards or published policies.
- Accreditation Withdrawn—program fails to comply with the Accreditation Standards or published policies within a specified time period.

The DPD provides the required dietetics coursework leading to a bachelor's or graduate degree. Graduates of ACEND-accredited programs who are verified by the program director may apply for Dietetic Internships to establish eligibility to write the CDR registration examination for dietitians.

For information on a specific program, contact the program director.

Search for programs

State: All States   Go   ☐ Only Programs Offering Distance Education
                                      ☐ Only Programs with Course Credit Transfer Agreements
                                      ☐ Only Programs that Result in a Graduate Degree
                                      ☐ Only Programs that have an ISPP option available

The information in this listing, including program details, is intended to be as accurate as possible when posted, but is subject to change without notice. The Academy of Nutrition and Dietetics and the Accreditation Council for Education in Nutrition and Dietetics assume no responsibility for changes or errors in the compilation of this information, and no one accessing and using the information shall have any right of recovery on account of its use.

The Career Change: Advanced Degree Programs

For career changers who have a bachelor's degree in an area other than dietetics and wish to become an RDN, one option is to pursue a graduate-level CP that includes both the didactic course work and supervised practice hours necessary to sit for the registration exam. There are also programs that allow students to complete the required didactic course work, after which they can apply for DIs (some are combined with a master's degree). Both pathways lead to the same outcome. Factors such as program emphasis, location, cost, timing, and other unique attributes will help you decide what is best for you. For more tips, see the following section on "Finding Your Best Program."

OTHER TIPS FOR CAREER CHANGERS

- **Working while going to school?** Consider looking into tuition reimbursement from your current job. As a part-time student, you may want to limit your course load to one to two courses per semester, as each hour of class time may require one to three hours of work outside of class.

- **Coming from a nonscience background?** Be encouraged by the fact that many RDNs started in another field and have successfully excelled in the sciences. Ask your program director to put you in touch with former students who made the switch, and get their take on how to navigate the challenges. Expect a heavy load of the life sciences. Although this can be challenging, this course work is fundamental to building an understanding of nutrition and human health.

- **Be prepared.** A positive attitude, efficient study skills, access to a tutor or study groups, and a commitment to succeed will help you make it through the more challenging aspects of the academic requirements.

Finding Your Best Program

As you consider the academic pathway that is best for you, there are also practical, personal, and professional considerations to take into account when researching and selecting a potential undergraduate and/or graduate program in nutrition and dietetics:

- What area of practice do you want to pursue? Whether you're interested in clinical, private, community, foodservice, or research practice (to name just a few) different programs can vary in their emphasis or concentration within dietetics and nutrition. This information can typically be found on the program's website, along with details about possible minors or unique opportunities.

- Do you have a specific preference for a geographic location? The city and state in which you study are important professional considerations since they will influence the work and volunteer opportunities available to you (eg, working with a farmers market in a rural setting versus leading nutrition classes for schools in a large city). Also consider your personal preference in terms of where you might live after academic study, as many job opportunities stem from experiences and connections fostered as a student or dietetic intern.
- What's the pace and personality of the department? Perspectives from students and faculty offer firsthand insights into a program. It's a good idea to visit prospective programs and speak to students in the programs.
- What does your gut say? In the end, only you can decide if a program feels right, and doing this legwork will help you make an informed choice. The ideal choice should match your interests, build on your strengths, and bolster your weaknesses.

Looking to the Future: New Educational Standards

As an accrediting agency, ACEND reviews its standards every five years for educational preparation for nutrition and dietetics practitioners. In its latest review, summarized in a 2015 report called *Rationale for Future Education Preparation for Nutrition and Dietetics Practitioners*, ACEND conducted an environmental scan and gathered input from key stakeholders regarding the future vision of dietetics practice.[3] Based on this research, ACEND recommended "a new model of education that includes moving the educational preparation of entry-level generalist dietitian nutritionists to the minimum of *master's level* [emphasis added]" and "moving the educational preparation of entry-level nutrition and dietetics technicians to the minimum of bachelor's level."[4] Raising the educational requirements will better prepare dietetics practitioners for the complex and diverse practice expectations of the future. It also reflects the expanding interest in and need for qualified nutrition and dietetics professionals. The standards and competencies for the future model of master's

A Closer Look

Highlighting Unique Nutrition Programs

The following examples highlight ACEND-accredited academic opportunities with a few unique specialty areas and approaches. These are just a few among many programs offered in the United States.

CULINARY NUTRITION PROGRAMS

Johnson & Wales University: Johnson & Wales was the first school to offer bachelors' degrees in culinary arts and baking and pastry arts. It was also the first to offer a bachelor of science in culinary nutrition—a hands-on culinary nutrition degree, accredited by ACEND, designed for students who seek to apply nutrition and food science principles to the culinary arts. Courses are taught by professional chefs and RDNs. The goal is to impart the technical and cognitive skills required of a self-reliant professional who can do the following: (1) manage the delivery of nutrition services to diverse populations and supervise daily operations of a food-service facility; (2) incorporate current nutrition theory into classic cuisine; (3) assure that operations meet the food and nutrition needs of clients; and (4) participate in activities that promote nutrition and the profession. More information about the culinary nutrition program is on the Johnson & Wales University website (https://academics.jwu.edu/college-of -culinary-arts/culinary-nutrition-bs/).

Saint Louis University—Culinary Arts Emphasis: Saint Louis University also offers a special emphasis in culinary arts for students within its nutrition and dietetics degree program that allows students to complete requirements for becoming an RDN and certified culinarian. In this emphasis, students learn culinary technique in modern food labs and "real-life" dining facilities, such as its Fresh Gatherings Cafe, which is run entirely by the nutrition and dietetics students. In general, the program takes a comprehensive approach, exposing students to complementary fields, such as food innovation and entrepreneurship (an additional special emphasis), sustainable food systems, and food science. Graduates of the program have a well-rounded viewpoint in preparation for a variety of food and health careers. Learn more about the major in nutrition and dietetics at the Saint Louis University website (www.slu.edu/nutrition-and-dietetics-x12857).

CONTINUED ›

A CLOSER LOOK (CONTINUED)   ....[5]

DISTANCE AND ONLINE DIDACTIC PROGRAM OPTIONS

University of Alabama, University of Northern Colorado, and Kansas State University: These three universities are among the programs that currently offer a distance or online DPD. These programs are designed to allow students in other geographical locations or with employment or family commitments to have access to the same resources and course work as if they were located on campus. At the University of Alabama, for example, the distance courses are all available online or via DVD. There are certain limitations, however, for students residing in certain states due to federal regulations. More information can be found directly from the program websites:

Alabama (www.nhm.ches.ua.edu/distance-education.html)

Northern Colorado (www.unco.edu/ddp/)

Kansas State (www.he.k-state.edu/hmd/ugrad/distance-dietetics/)

MULTICULTURAL EMPHASIS

Spanish Emphasis at Marywood University: Marywood University in Pennsylvania offers a Spanish-emphasis option for dietetics students. In this program, students complete the course work for a Spanish minor in addition to the DPD requirements and have the unique opportunity to study abroad in a Latin American country for a portion of one semester. The program is planned in such a way that students still graduate in the same amount of time as they would in a traditional DPD. Given the cultural diversity

level dietitian nutritionist programs are expected to be released in 2017. Additional details and updates, including frequently asked questions and suggestions to improve your chances of being accepted into a dietetic internship, can be found on the ACEND website.[5]

As a credentialing agency, the Commission on Dietetic Registration (CDR) also routinely reviews its requirements for credentials it offers for nutrition and dietetics practitioners. Based on data collected for the *Council on Future Practice Visioning Report*, CDR changed the education eligibility requirements for the dietitian registration examination to a minimum of a master's degree effective January 1, 2024.

in the United States, such an emphasis can be invaluable in developing students as a more effective service provider. Details are on the Marywood University website (www.marywood.edu/nutrition/undergraduate -programs/didactic/).

Multicultural Scholars in Dietetics Program (MSDP) at the University of North Dakota: The MSDP was inspired by a need for care providers to understand the cultural context of food, nutrition, and health choices. It focuses especially on increasing the proportion of American Indian, Alaska Native, or Hawaiian Native dietetics practitioners. The MSDP aims to recruit highly qualified American Indian scholars who are interested in becoming RDNs and then assisting these individuals academically as well as financially (through financial scholarship) in reaching their potential. For more information, visit the MSDP website (http://nursing .und.edu/departments/nutrition-dietetics/msdp.cfm).

SPORTS NUTRITION OPPORTUNITIES DURING THE DIDACTIC PROGRAM

Many academic programs offer sports nutrition course work to dietetics students. For example, Florida State University's dietetics program includes the DPD course work and provides students the opportunity to take introductory sports nutrition classes. Additional programs with an emphasis on sports nutrition are found on the Sports, Cardiovascular, and Wellness Nutrition (SCAN) dietetic practice group website (www.scandpg .org/sports-nutrition-education-programs).

Your Degree Options

In dietetics and nutrition, your degrees and credentials demonstrate to patients and clients that you've earned the right to care for them and provide nutrition services. After high school, undergraduate programs grant bachelor's degrees, typically a bachelor of science (BS) for nutritional sciences or a bachelor of arts (BA). Currently, at least a bachelor's degree is necessary to become an RDN. An ACEND-accredited DPD can also be completed while an undergraduate, before entering a DI. Although different advanced degrees may be associated with varying salary ranges, attaining an advanced degree can help open the door for more opportunities.

Master's Degrees in Nutrition : MS, MA, MEd

Completing a master's degree is an increasingly important consideration, as we mentioned previously in "Looking to the Future: New Educational Standards." Master's degrees, such as a master of science (MS) or master of arts (MA), require advanced course work and training, and they prepare graduates for more specialized or advanced nutrition-related positions in clinical, management, administration, and research specialties. Some master's degree students may already be RDNs; others may be career changers who are simultaneously working toward completing a DPD, DI, and graduate degree. The specific requirements may vary by program and may require students to complete a research thesis, comprehensive exam, or culminating project. A master's degree in education (MEd) emphasizes health or nutrition education. Graduates of these programs are qualified for a number of roles, including curriculum development, policy advisement, health care, research, and academia.

Complementary Master's Degrees: MPH, MBA

In addition to the degrees mentioned, dietetics students may also be interested in master's degrees in public health (MPH) or business administration (management) (MBA). Both degrees are related to the field of nutrition and dietetics, depending on your specialty area of practice. An MPH prepares a student to work in community health and nutrition, research, administration, and public policy development, while an MBA cultivates expertise in business, management, economics, and human resources, among other areas.

Doctoral Degrees: PhD, DrPH, ScD, EdD, DCN

A doctor of philosophy (PhD) is the more common doctoral degree, but there are also doctorates in public health (DrPH), science (ScD), and education (EdD). As the highest level of education, these programs, called terminal degrees, are a large commitment, requiring graduate course work, independent research, completion of comprehensive exams, and a dissertation. A nutrition PhD is suited for individuals pursuing research or careers in academia. For advanced clinical training and evidence-based practice skills, the Rutgers School of Health Related Professions in New Jersey offers a doctor of clinical nutrition (DCN) degree, which requires a clinical residency as well as a research project.

For doctoral degree holders who are not RDNs and do not have a DPD verification statement, the new individualized supervised practice pathway (ISPP), covered in Chapter 3, can offer an alternative supervised practice option. With their advanced training and experience in areas such as research, these self-directed individuals can pursue ISPPs in order to have time to complete the competencies on a more flexible, independent, or part-time schedule, if needed.

Out of the Classroom and into the Real World (Kind Of)

It is important for nutrition and dietetics students to get real-world experience outside of the classroom. Fieldwork, independent study, volunteering, and summer internships are all great ways to get this experience while earning money and receiving academic credit. It's a change of pace from traditional course work and also helps with discovering your professional likes and, just as important, dislikes. Real-world experience also helps make you well-rounded. You'll learn skills that are transferable to other settings—the classroom, a dietetic internship, and future jobs. You'll also demonstrate your ability to plan ahead and manage your time by balancing these additional time commitments with course work. Finally, it's an opportunity to make valuable contacts for future recommendation letters, career advice, or mentorships.

Before you embark on any of these experiences, evaluate your current status as a student. How much time can you reasonably commit to nonclassroom activities? If you are too busy during the school year, maybe a summer internship is more appropriate. In what type of environment do you thrive—a bustling public health clinic or a quiet medical laboratory? Can you work a demanding schedule and take on greater responsibilities? Answering these questions will help you focus your efforts most efficiently.

Fieldwork, Independent Study, and Assistantships

In addition to excelling as a student, you can enrich your educational experience through nutrition-related fieldwork or independent study done concurrently with classes.

Fieldwork allows students to integrate and apply academic knowledge and skills at progressively higher levels of performance and responsibility. The student gains work experience while carrying out projects that contribute to professional growth. Some academic programs include mandatory fieldwork for credit (for example, volunteering at a local soup kitchen during a community nutrition course). Even if not required, fieldwork experience is recommended because it lets you apply what you learned in the classroom to the real world. This may focus on wellness, public health, foodservice management, nutrition in ambulatory care, home health care, or clinical services.

Independent study is another structured way to gain experience beyond your didactic program, allowing you the chance to explore academic topics outside of your standard courses. For example, you could arrange with an instructor to independently study an area of dietetics that interests you and complete a summary project of your findings. Alternatively, you may seek research experience by working in a professor's laboratory as a research assistant. Some schools have honors research programs through which you can conduct your own study and complete a thesis paper.

Teaching assistantships are available at certain schools and programs, either for academic credit or payment. These programs allow students, typically juniors and seniors, to work within a teaching team for a course they have taken already. These are typically more introductory courses, but they will offer a great opportunity to improve your leadership skills, hone your knowledge of the course materials, and gain experience educating others.

Ultimately, taking initiative to gain this experience will show your commitment to the field and your "go-getter" mentality when you apply for the dietetic internship and future jobs.

Volunteering

An unwritten rule in dietetics is the importance of volunteering your time. It shows you have an interest in the community and provides a way to practice your talents and learn new skills. Don't worry if you're not working directly with an RDN. Any experience counts— especially if you are giving valuable time to a worthy cause. If you can work with other nutrition or health professionals, such as in a hospital or health care setting, seize this opportunity. Start by shadowing registered dietitians as they work with clients. Then, look for ways to apply your nutrition knowledge, such as by volunteering to create educational materials for a local hospital, clinic, or health club.

If you feel unsure where to start, speak with a professor, adviser, or program director—they can provide advice and contacts to pursue. Consider working within health departments; nutrition education programs; hunger relief or food assistance programs, such as a food bank or the government-sponsored Special Supplemental Nutrition Program for Women, Infants, and Children (WIC); farmers markets; or family resource centers.

Summer Internships

By summer internship, we refer to an optional work experience that students may take between semesters—not to be confused with the structured ACEND-accredited dietetic internship that fulfills the supervised practice criteria. Although previously the summer was a time to relax and take off from school, the reality is that most working adults do not have the entire summer off for vacation. A summer internship is an investment in your future. Utilizing the summer months to get work experience through a nutrition- or food-related internship will give you the chance to (1) spend an extended period of time immersed in a project; (2) contribute meaningful work to a company, hospital, or other facility; and (3) begin to network and meet contacts for the future.

Don't know where you want to work? Start by tapping the resources available to you. What's accessible on campus? Is there a medical center, community clinic, or student health service where you can gain experience? University foodservice operations also have food-related work experiences available to students. Your college's career center will have advice for job opportunities on and off campus, suggest alumni who might be hiring, and offer tips for resume writing and interviewing skills for when you apply.

What about opportunities in the surrounding community, neighboring cities, back home, or in new cities? Other resources for jobs might be long-term-care facilities (such as nursing homes and assisted-living facilities), hospices, adult and pediatric daycare facilities, or government health departments or other community programs. Even waiting tables or working in food retail can be applicable experiences to learn about foodservice operations and safe food handling. Once you have your eye on specific opportunities, take the following steps:

- Contact the facility or organization.
- Ask if they are hiring or taking on volunteers. Many facilities and organizations are eager to accept students.
- Consult with your program adviser to brainstorm goals to accomplish during your experience.

Send out resumes with a cover letter describing who you are, your special skills, and what you hope to contribute and learn from the experience. Persistence is key.

Take-Home Tips: Going Above and Beyond

In the next chapter, we'll discuss the process of applying for and matching to a DI, which has become very competitive over recent years. It's therefore critical that you do everything possible while completing the DPD to make your application shine. The following tips can help you stand out and increase the likelihood of your success[6]:

SELECTED VOLUNTEER ORGANIZATIONS

- United Way
- American Cancer Society
- Red Cross
- Local health departments
- Food banks
- WIC
- VolunteerMatch.org

- Idealist.org
- LinkedIn for Volunteers (https://volunteer.linkedin.com)
- HandsOn Network (www.handsonnetwork.org)
- Dosomething.org

- Make sure your GPA is above the minimum required by potential internships. It's true that GPA is not the only factor considered, but it is one of the most highly weighted. A GPA of 3.0 is often the minimum, but chances are that applicants with a higher GPA will be more competitive. The same principles apply for GRE scores, if applicable.
- Volunteer and provide community service, especially in areas related to health and nutrition. If possible, volunteer at a facility that serves as a practice site for an internship program so that preceptors and the program director can become familiar with you and your abilities.
- Get practical, paid work experiences, especially related to your desired area(s) of practice.
- Get involved (especially in leadership roles) in professional organizations, such as college dietetics clubs and district, state, and national nutrition and dietetics associations.
- Publish and present any relevant research, projects, or work that you have done in journals, at conferences, or in poster sessions.

References

1. Accreditation Council for Education in Nutrition and Dietetics. Frequently asked questions about careers in dietetics. http://www.eatrightacend.org/ACEND/content.aspx?id=6442485476. Published April 2015. Accessed January 17, 2016.

2. Accreditation Council for Education in Nutrition and Dietetics. Didactic programs in dietetics. http://www.eatrightacend.org /ACEND/content.aspx?id=6442485422. Accessed January 10, 2016.

3. Accreditation Council for Education in Nutrition and Dietetics. *Rationale for Future Education Preparation of Nutrition and Dietetics Practitioners.* http://www.eatrightacend.org/WorkArea /linkit.aspx?LinkIdentifier=id&ItemID=6442486380&libID =6442486356. Updated August 2015. Accessed January 10, 2016.

4. Accreditation Council for Education in Nutrition and Dietetics. ACEND Standards Committee. http://www.eatrightacend.org /ACEND/content.aspx?id=6442485290. Accessed January 10, 2016.

5. Accreditation Council for Education in Nutrition and Dietetics. Suggestions to improve your chances at getting a dietetic-internship position: student guidance document. http://www.eatrightacend .org/ACEND/content.aspx?id=6442485432. Updated August 1, 2009. Accessed January 10, 2016.

CHAPTER 3

The Match: Applying to Dietetic Internships

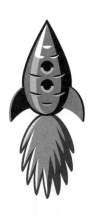

THOUGHT QUESTIONS

- Research a few dietetic internship programs that appeal to you. Why did you choose them? Any criteria or reason is allowed.

- Do these programs have specific requirements different from other programs for the dietetic internship application process?

- Create a detailed list of everything you will need and the steps you'll have to take to apply to one of these programs.

THE NEXT MAJOR MILESTONE IN YOUR JOURNEY TO BE-coming a registered dietitian nutritionist (RDN) is the super-vised practice component, also called the dietetic internship (DI). It comes after you've fulfilled the didactic program in dietetics (DPD) requirements (covered in Chapter 2) but before taking the credentialing exam. All students completing the DPD must apply to an Accreditation Council for Education in Nutrition and Dietetics (ACEND)–accredited dietetic internship to complete their dietetics training. Remember that coordinated programs (CPs) in dietetics combine the didactic course work and supervised experience in one program, allowing you to forego the process of applying to DIs.

Dietetic Internships: A to Z

In 2015, there were more than 250 ACEND-accredited DIs, each with unique emphases and features. Some are traditional DI-only programs that take about 8 to 12 months to complete. Others are combined mas-ter's/DI programs that require graduate course work in addition to supervised practice. These programs typically take two years and result in a graduate degree. Other dietetics programs have an indi-vidualized supervised practice pathway (ISPP) option, an alternate supervised practice option for motivated students who (1) graduated from an accredited DPD program and did not match to a DI but have obtained a verification statement or (2) hold a doctoral degree but have not completed the DPD or obtained a verification statement.

Even with all of these options, being accepted into a DI is an in-creasingly competitive process. Over recent years, the match rate has averaged about 50%, due to a high volume of applicants. For example, data from 2015 show that there were 3,158 DI openings and 5,853 applicants, resulting in 54% match potential.[1]

That's why we're here to help! This chapter will provide an over-view of the DI application process: suggestions for finding the right DI; an outline of steps involved in the application process, including "the match"; and tips for putting together a winning application and interview experience. Chapter 4, "What You Need to Know About Di-etetic Internships," offers details about the DI *after* you are accepted.

Getting Ready to Apply

According to current ACEND standards, before you can apply for a dietetic internship, you must complete an ACEND-accredited DPD. This is a structured dietetics curriculum that results in a bachelor's degree. During the application process, you will need to submit either a declaration of intent to complete form or a verification statement to verify your completion of (or intent to complete) the DPD requirements. You will also need to submit an official copy of your transcript from your college or university to verify your bachelor's degree (see Figure 3.1).

FIGURE 3.1.
Paperwork you'll need for dietetic internship applications

Declaration of Intent to Complete:	Verification Statement:	Official Transcript:
• Submitted with applications if DPD and/ or bachelor's degree is not yet complete • Signed and dated by DPD	• Submitted after your bachelor's degree is conferred by your university or college and DPD course work has been completed	• Obtained from your college or university registrar • Provides an official summary of the courses you've taken and

The declaration of intent form is needed by DI applicants who are still in school. Because you haven't finished the DPD course work yet, this form will be included in your DI application and declares that you intend to complete your course work before the internship would begin. Your director will sign the form, based on a review of your transcripts mid-semester.

The verification statement is completed upon graduation with a bachelor's degree and completion of the DPD course work. This is also completed by your director, pending an evaluation of your transcript and a confirmation that you are approved for and in good standing for graduation. Do not lose this verification statement! Your director will give you at least six originals; you will give one to your DI and will likely need others in the future for the state licensing board, graduate school, or an employer.

While getting this paperwork in order, you should also begin to research the many different programs. (See the next section, Researching the Dietetic Internship.) After you find a few that you are interested in, the best way to find out more is by contacting and, if possible, visiting individual programs directly—this also shows great initiative and provides reviewers with a face to match the name when your application comes through.

Researching the Dietetic Internship

Similar to the online resource mentioned in Chapter 2 for researching DPD programs, the Academy of Nutrition and Dietetics and ACEND also offer a useful online resource for sorting and exploring the different accredited dietetic internships across the country.[2] Use this tool to do the following:

- Look up programs by state and determine whether they offer distance education and whether they result in a graduate degree or have an ISPP option.
- Find links to program websites to learn more details or plan a visit.
- Learn about the program's department and area of concentration (such as public health, management, nutrition therapy, research, education, and more).
- Obtain important details, including
    - > the name and contact information of the program director;
    - > the annual enrollment size, timing, and length of the program;
    - > the program cost, in terms of tuition, fees, stipends, and financial aid;
    - > timing for the match and application deadlines; and
    - > accreditation status, which will be candidacy for accreditation, accredited, probationary accreditation, or accreditation withdrawn.

A Closer Look

Finding the Right Internship for You

This following insights are from an application coach's perspective. Kyle and Milton interviewed Jenny Westerkamp, RD, owner of All Access Internships (www.allaccessinternships.com).

Kyle and Milton: As founder of All Access Internships, a resource for aspiring RDNs, what is the most important thing an applicant needs to know about the DI?

Jenny: The dietetic internship is the transition between student and professional. We are lucky to have this time to evolve without having to dive right into a career. As both a student and professional, interns will have projects and homework assignments on top of clocking in from at least 9 to 5. Balance will be a running theme throughout the internship— balancing work, assignments, your health, and fun, too! Overall, it's an experience that will help you grow both personally and professionally and prepare you well for the real world.

K & M: What's your advice on what to consider when looking for a good DI match?

Jenny: Many factors differentiate internship programs. These include location, expense, emphasis, length, rotation locations, elective rotation options, graduate credit options, or distance internship options, to name a few. Consider what you can realistically afford to do, and choose from programs that match your interests and experiences. I was willing to look across the country for internships. I knew I wanted a well-rounded emphasis, was attracted to teaching hospitals, and wanted the option to do an elective rotation in a specialty or location of my choice. Massachusetts General Hospital offered all of that, and that is where I matched. When you apply to programs that fit your interests, a genuine enthusiasm for the program will shine through to the selection committee and will reflect well on your application. The "match" works two ways—both you and the program should fit well with each other. Proving you are the perfect fit is what the application is for!

K & M: What's the best way for the DI applicant to evaluate a program?

Jenny: Learn about the program's rotations and the level of responsibility you will have at these rotation sites. Are rotation sites accustomed to

CONTINUED ›

A CLOSER LOOK (CONTINUED)

having interns? Will you be mostly observing or mostly participating in tasks? Talk with former or current interns about their experiences (both the pros and the cons of the program). Decide if the internship culture is attractive to you (that is, the director's work style, department culture, and institution culture). Of course, make sure that your GPA and resume of experience is competitive with that of the current interns who have been matched.

K & M: Is there a magic number for how many an applicant should apply to?

Jenny: When applying to programs with computer matching, your chances of acceptance by these programs will vary based on your rankings. It is impossible to accurately predict the effect that ranking a program will have on your chances, as this is also dependent on how many people apply to those programs and rank the programs higher. In general, four to five programs is a good recommendation. I typically observe that students get into one of their top three choices or get no match at all.

K & M: Do you have any recommendations for networking with other interns or applicants?

Jenny: All Access Internships has an always expanding collection of resources for this purpose, including our Facebook Group, Dietetics Student Support Group. It's also fair to ask the dietetic internship directors of the programs you are interested in to introduce you to current interns or ask your didactic program director for contact information of alumni.

K & M: Anything else you wish to add?

Jenny: My best advice for excelling in the application process and internship is summed up in this quote by John Wooden: "Things turn out best for the people who make the best of the way things turn out." No matter what happens on the road to becoming an RDN (the stress of the application process and the challenges that come before you are in the internship), having a positive attitude every step of the way will be one of the most important keys to your success as a student, intern, *and* registered dietitian!

The Fine Print: The Dietetic Internship Application

Once you have spent time looking into potential programs and deciding what is right for you, it's time to put together your application. There are two main steps required for the dietetic internship application process.

1. The Dietetic Internship Centralized Application System (DICAS) Application: Most DI programs allow you to apply using a more efficient, common online application called DICAS (http://portal.dicas.org/). Implemented in 2010, DICAS now allows prospective dietetic interns to complete one application, submit one set of transcripts, and pay program fees electronically to cover all application costs instead of applying to individual programs separately. Some programs still require a separate or written application, but most have moved to DICAS.

2. D&D Digital Computer Matching: In addition to submitting your applications through DICAS, there is a separate online system administered by D&D Digital that you must register with for the "computer match" (www.dnddigital.com/ada /index.php). In this second step, prospective interns are asked to rank the programs they apply to. Similarly, DI programs use D&D Digital to rank a priority list of applicants. The computer will then "match" each applicant to the highest-ranking program that offers that applicant a position. To be clear, each applicant is matched with only one program, which the applicant can accept or decline. The very few programs that do not participate in the matching process will accept applications under different circumstances.

This all may sound complicated, but fortunately there are resources to help. Your program director, if you are enrolled in a DPD, will be there to provide guidance when the time comes. It is *very* important to visit the website of all the programs you are considering to confirm the application materials they require. Additionally, DICAS and D&D Digital both offer instructions, FAQs, and other resources to help applicants navigate the steps.

Staying on Track: An Applicant's Timeline and Overview

Here is a list of tips to help you make your way through the DI application process.

1. Start early and give yourself enough time to complete your applications on time. Typically, applications for the spring match are due in early February for internships beginning the following summer or fall, but some programs have earlier deadlines in January. A few DIs also participate in the fall match, which takes place in November, but this is less common. We recommend beginning the applications at least three to four months before the deadline and setting aside enough time to complete strong applications without any errors or typos. Internship directors will pay attention to such details.

2. Check the application requirements for each internship program. Does it use DICAS? Are there any other unique requirements, such as submitting an additional essay? When applying to multiple internships, develop a system for keeping the information pertaining to each school separate to avoid any confusion.

3. Take the Graduate Record Examination (GRE; www.ets.org /gre) if you're applying to graduate degree programs that require it. Allow plenty of time to sit for the GRE at least once, if not more than once, and for your scores to be processed.

4. Complete the DICAS or other application. This will ask for your contact information and background, your DPD program contact information, and your educational information and academic performance, especially in the DPD courses. You may also list any awards or honors, professional experiences, and volunteer activities.

5. Include your personal statement. This writing sample is required for all applicants and asks you to address the following thought questions: Why do you want to enter the dietetics

profession? What experiences have helped prepare you for your career? What are your short-term and long-term goals? What are your strengths and weaknesses? What other information do you consider important for the selection decision? We suggest drafting the personal statement well in advance to allow time for edits; keep track of the character limit. Other program-specific writing topics may be responses to specific questions about ethical dilemmas, clinical nutrition, food science, work-related scenarios, and so forth.

6. Obtain and submit the declaration of intent to complete or the verification statement, described earlier in the chapter, from your DPD program director, depending on your status as a dietetics student at the time of your application.

7. Upload a resume that details your educational background, work, and volunteer experience. This may summarize much of the information elsewhere in your application. Your college or university's career center, DPD director, or other professors/mentors can be helpful resume reviewers.

8. Secure strong references or letters of recommendation. Consider your academic adviser, professors, DPD director, or previous employer or supervisor. Ask potential reference providers if they have the time and if they are comfortable with writing you a glowing recommendation. It's best if you ask as far in advance as possible since these individuals are quite busy. Also be prepared to provide details about yourself, such as a resume, and suggestions for your strengths and experiences that they might highlight.

Send official transcripts to DICAS from each school you attended. This can often take a few weeks, especially around the winter holidays, which is why it is a good idea to use a calendar to plan ahead and stay on track.

Register for computer matching with D&D Digital. D&D Digital is the online service that facilitates the process. Remember that because each applicant is matched with only one program it's extremely

PAPERWORK FOR INTERNATIONAL STUDENTS

There are special requirements for students whose bachelor's or master's degree is from a college or university outside of the United States. Visit the "International Students" section within the Student Center of the Academy's website for more information.[3]

OTHER COMMON Q&A FOR DIETETIC INTERNSHIP APPLICANTS

How many should I apply to? Some students apply to only one DI, while others apply to 10. Both approaches are extreme. Shooting for only one program reduces your chances of getting an appointment, while going for 10 is very expensive. Instead, pick a happy medium. Apply to a range of programs to cover your bases, but apply only to those you would be satisfied to attend. If matched, you will only have the opportunity to work with one program, so ask your program director to develop a varied but reasonable list of programs based on your interest, experiences, and career goals.

Should I plan to visit the programs? We highly recommend visiting the top programs on your list the semester or season before you plan to apply. This provides an opportunity to meet the director, tour the facility, and get an in-person feel for whether the program is the right fit. This *may* boost your chances of getting in. Alternatively, you might discover that the program isn't right for you. Some programs have formal open house events that you can attend; others have regularly scheduled tour days. Be on your toes the whole time, since some tours also act as informal interviews. Remember that although a visit won't guarantee admission, there are plenty of advantages—both for you and the program.

Is there any strategy to ranking programs? Ranking should be taken very seriously. It's best to put your number-one choice first. Be confident in yourself, but also apply to a range of programs, including at least one that you feel you have a good likelihood of being accepted into. Your program director is a good resource for judging your chances since he or she will have experience seeing applicants get matched. It is important to consider your priorities and how your qualifications compare to those of applicants accepted in previous years.

important to apply only to internships with which you would be willing to accept an appointment.

Final Thoughts on the Application

Your dietetic internship application is your life story condensed into an online template. Through your personal statement, letters of reference, extracurricular activities, honors and awards, grades, paid work experiences, volunteer activities, and course work, the dietetic internship programs will learn of your capabilities and personality and decide if you would be a good fit for their department. The standardized application is accepted by many programs, but remember that some schools may use their own applications or ask for supplemental information. Do not let that confuse you. Focus on reading the instructions for each school and then following them closely.

Proofreading

A WORD ABOUT GRADES

Although your application will be evaluated in its entirety, grades from college and graduate school are an important factor. Having good scores helps boost your chances of getting an appointment. But, if you have below-average grades, we recommend addressing the issue, perhaps in an interview or in the personal statement. Explain why you struggled: Maybe you were still developing time-management skills, or perhaps living in the dormitory was too distracting. Then explain how you fixed this: You started keeping a personal organizer or spent more time studying in the library. Use your subsequent grades to substantiate any claims and reassure committee members that you plan to excel in their demanding program.

When you are finished with your application, triple-check everything! Make sure there are no typos or grammatical errors. Ask a friend, ideally a good critic, to proofread your application materials. You may even offer to pay your critic to inspire true proofreading. Some folks accidentally send applications or letters to the wrong schools. As you can imagine, this does not leave a good impression!

A Closer Look

Internship Director's Corner

This section features an interview with Karen Wetherall, MS, RDN, LDN, the dietetic internship director at the University of Tennessee (UT) Knoxville.

Kyle and Milton: From your perspective as an internship director, what is the most important thing student applicants need to know about dietetic internships?

Karen: All accredited internships provide experiences related to the basic areas of practice to meet all ACEND competencies. Hence, students will get what they need to practice in dietetics and to pass the RD exam, no matter the internship. However, internships design their programs utilizing specific strengths and local resources. For example, the master's degree program at UT, Knoxville has a public health nutrition track. In addition to clinical rotations, we have a strong network of community and public health sites and preceptors incorporated into our internship experience. Program directors, including myself, encourage applicants to identify programs that align with their areas of interest. Do realize that some interests—like sports nutrition, eating disorders, or neonatal nutrition—are beyond entry-level, and experience after the internship is likely necessary to specialize in these areas.

K & M: Is there something that would help students rank more favorably when applying to internships?

Karen: Students should be working to obtain the highest GPA and GRE scores as possible. Those are the baseline criteria. Programs also value a well-rounded resume, so those applicants with a lower GPA would especially want to highlight their work and leadership experience. At our program, we appreciate both paid and volunteer experience. We like to see some clinical experience (even if it's just shadowing RDNs) along with some other nutrition-related experience (for example, nutrition education through after-school programs, camps, health fairs). We suggest 500 hours of work and leadership experience.

Beyond that, the personal statement is a wonderful tool to market a student's application. Program directors have stated that this letter can really set an applicant apart, along with letters of recommendation that speak on behalf of the individual. Hopefully these letters strengthen an application. The person providing the reference should be a faculty member who knows the applicant's school performance or an RDN who knows the applicant's work performance. Periodically we'll receive references from the applicant's neighbor who is also a dean or from a graduate assistant the applicant worked for at a fitness facility. These are not the strongest, nor the most professional choices for references.

K & M: Think about the top applicants you have admitted to your internship program. What stands out most about them?

Karen: I'm looking for a balanced applicant. What does that mean? Strong grades, with a GPA of 3.4 or higher, a variety of quality work experience and additional leadership experience (perhaps a board position in a sorority or nutrition organization), and supportive, favorable recommendations. Their personal statement would reflect both passion and drive for learning in the field of nutrition and a desire to make a difference. Some top applicants had experience above and beyond expectations, such as travel abroad studying food culture or working with children on a mission project. Others may have gone the extra mile by being in an honors program and having participated in undergraduate research. Finally, a reference letter that states, "This is one of the top five students I have worked with in my 15-year career" (for example) speaks volumes for the applicant.

K & M: Anything else you wish to add?

Karen: In summary, students should work to obtain a variety of experiences, create positive relationships with faculty and mentors, and take time to create a well-written, error-free personal statement. That statement should reflect their love for the field, speak to the strengths and skills they've developed during their life experience, and address interest areas, including some possible future plans once they've obtained their RDN.

The student should also address why the program is of interest and is a good fit, because after all, the student and program should be a good match! Study the website of each program and follow specific guidelines for each application. Most internship directors welcome an e-mail indicating

CONTINUED ›

A CLOSER LOOK (CONTINUED) ··

interest in their program. Many programs have an open house, or the direc-tor may set up individual appointments for students to visit at their conve-nience. Whenever possible, travel to these events to further research the program. It's not too early to begin researching and visiting programs in the junior year. It's also not too early to begin the application process by visit-ing the DICAS website in the fall and asking for letters of recommendation from faculty and mentors at least a month before they are needed. Having more time to write a recommendation will result in the better outcome!

The Interview

Many dietetic internships require an interview. If a program requests an interview, this means the committee is interested in you as a can-didate and wants to further compare you to other top candidates. To prepare, pull together work samples and your resume, research the program and its faculty extensively, and take time to practice your answers to potential questions. Consider creating an online portfolio or putting samples on a flash drive for your interview.

The interview could go in a number of different directions, but it is likely to begin with "So, tell us a little bit about yourself." This request allows you two minutes or less to tell the interviewer your life story. Hit the high points: education, achievements, background, and where you're headed. Be prepared to speak about your strengths and weaknesses, and try to turn your weaknesses into something positive. Finally, practice aloud with a friend—nailing this exercise will pave the way for a smooth interview.

Remember, interviewing is intense for both the candidates and the interviewers, so do not be surprised if interviews are shorter than you expect. Answer questions fully and confidently, be comfort-able pausing for a few seconds after a tough question to gather your thoughts, and come in prepared with your own questions.

FIGURE 3.2.
Final review: steps for applying to dietetic internships

Research and identify the DIs that interest you most.

- This should be determined from the internship type, concentration, availability of graduate study, location, cost, financial aid, class size, and any other unique features that may apply.

Visit the top DI that you are interested in.

- Most programs will host either an open house or regular tours. Certain ones require you to make an appointment in order to attend. If a visit is not possible, set up a phone call appointment with the program director in order to meet, express your interest in the program, and answer any questions you have.

Register with DICAS.

- Use this online application service, where you can upload all of your application materials and select which DI programs to submit your application to. It's an efficient system, and it comes with a fee dependent on the number of additional DIs you apply to.

Fill out and submit all necessary DICAS application information.

- Calculate your GPA based on the DPD courses you've taken.
- Request your DPD director submit the declaration of intent or verification statement form, depending on your status as a student.
- Check each dietetic internship to determine if any supplemental materials are required in addition to the standard DICAS application.

Register with D&D Digital for computer matching.

- D&D Digital is the separate online service that helps match applicants and dietetic internships. Note that D&D Digital does not change the selection process. A program will not obtain an applicant who is not on its priority list, and an applicant will not be matched to a program he or she did not rank. D&D Digital also requires a fee.

APPLICATION TIP: RESEARCH YOUR INTERVIEWERS! A student shared the following experience with us. Alex had a telephone interview with a program in Virginia. Before the interview, he rehearsed his two-minute drill, had an extra copy of his resume handy, and collected samples of some of his best work from school for easy reference.

Despite this and the preparation he did in the days before the interview, Alex still felt he could have done better. Why? He was on a conference call with five interviewers, and it was difficult to keep names and titles straight. The whole process was intimidating. The lesson: When you are asked for an interview—whether it's on the phone or in person—find out the number of participants and their names and titles in advance. You'll be better prepared the day of the interview.

References

1. Accreditation Council for Education in Nutrition and Dietetics. *ACEND UPdate* (online newsletter for ACEND-accredited programs). http://www.eatrightacend.org/ACEND/content.aspx?id=6442485505. Accessed January 12, 2016.

2. Accreditation Council for Education in Nutrition and Dietetics. Dietetic internships. http://eatrightacend.org/ACEND/content.aspx?id=6442485424. Accessed January 12, 2016.

3. Academy of Nutrition and Dietetics. Become an RDN or DTR: international students. http://www.eatrightpro.org/resources/career/become-an-rdn-or-dtr/international-students. Accessed January 12, 2016.

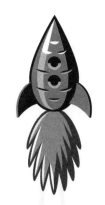

CHAPTER 4

What You Need to Know About Dietetic Internships

THOUGHT QUESTIONS

- What aspects are you most looking forward to during the internship experience? Explain why.

- If you have the opportunity in your future dietetic internship, name a few special or elective rotations that you might consider selecting.

- What do you think it takes to be a preceptor? Summarize the job description of a preceptor and important skills or attributes for being a good preceptor.

NOW THAT YOU'VE BEEN ACCEPTED INTO A DIETETIC internship (DI) program using our advice from the previous chapter, you might be wondering what you've gotten yourself into! This chapter will provide an overview of the DI, including its objectives, the different areas of emphasis or concentration, and your responsibilities as a dietetic intern. Financial aid considerations will also be covered.

Dietetic Internships 101

The DI is designed to prepare interns to meet the performance requirements for entry-level registered dietitian nutritionists (RDNs). So, what's it all about? Here is a summary of details you'll want to understand about DIs.

Accreditation

To become accredited, DI programs must be evaluated by the Accreditation Council for Education in Nutrition and Dietetics (ACEND) on a set of standard criteria relating to quality assurance, organizational structure, location, financial stability, the awarding of degrees or certificates, program length, and program management, among other factors. Programs must designate at least two goals that reflect a mission or vision and must have measurable objectives to evaluate the achievement of these goals. Such objectives will pertain to the RDN credentialing exam pass rate, employment outlook, and other outcomes among program graduates.[1]

Internship Length

Students must complete at least 1,200 hours of supervised practice to be eligible for the RDN credentialing exam. Most full-time DI-only programs last about 8 to 12 months. A combined DI/master's program will take longer, about two years, because you will need to complete additional graduate course work for the master's degree. Coordinated programs in dietetics, which integrate supervised practice with the didactic course work and completion of at least a bachelor's degree, will also require 1,200 hours of supervised practice over the course of the program, though the structure and timing may vary slightly from the internship-only programs.

Competencies

Part of accreditation is meeting the core competencies determined by ACEND. These competencies are the minimum requirements necessary for entry-level practice. It's important to note that these competencies, summarized in Figure 4.1, "Core competency areas," are different from the essential practice competencies discussed in Chapter 6, which are specific to continuing education to maintain your RDN credential. During accreditation review, DI programs must outline the learning activities that interns will be offered in each area in order to develop proficiency. Standardizing the curriculum in this way helps to ensure that program completion, regardless of the internship you choose, will have prepared you to pass the registration exam and perform as a respected, credentialed professional.

Figure 4.1 shows the core competency areas identified by ACEND standards for entry-level dietitians.[1,2] Each competency also has specific subobjectives (not summarized here).

FIGURE 4.1.
Core competency areas[1]

Scientific and Evidence Base of Practice: Integration of scientific information and research into practice	Professional Practice Expectations: Beliefs, values, attitudes, and behaviors for the professional dietitian level of practice	Clinical and Customer Services: Development and delivery of information, products, and services to individuals, groups, and populations

Practice Management and Use of Resources: Strategic application of principles of management and systems in the provision of services to individuals and organizations	Concentration Area or Specialty Emphasis: Development of additional skills and knowledge to practice within a designated emphasis

Concentrations

In addition to the core competencies, DIs also may have a concentration area—a designation that the program curriculum will provide the experience necessary to develop proficiency in that specialty practice area. According to ACEND's 2012 report *Accreditation Standards for Internship Programs in Nutrition and Dietetics*, "a program concentration is an area which the program does well and wants to teach to students. . . . [Concentration] should support the mission of the program and be compatible with it."[1] Programs can have more than one concentration. Examples of concentrations in various internship programs are provided later in this chapter.

Rotations

In order to meet these core competencies, the DI takes place as a series of "rotations," which are semi-independent, short-term experiences in health care, community, foodservice, and management settings, to name a few. Programs may differ slightly in the relative proportion of time spent in each specialty. For example, a DI with a concentration in clinical nutrition or medical nutrition therapy may have more rotations in the hospital providing acute inpatient care, while a concentration in public health will have more rotations in community-based settings. The types of rotations involved with each DI can be found on individual program websites. This should be an important factor in your internship selection, based on your career interests and where you hope to expand and apply your knowledge of dietetics. If you're not sure, it's a good idea to consider internships with more general concentrations.

Responsibilities

During supervised practice, dietetic interns work under the guidance of a preceptor, defined as a registered dietitian nutritionist or other professional who has the appropriate knowledge, experience, and credentialing/licensure (if applicable) in the area he or she is supervising. You will typically start off observing or shadowing your preceptor(s) and then take on greater responsibilities, demonstrating independence, as you go. In some cases, you will have projects to complete either before or after each rotation. This "homework" helps prepare you for the rotation and summarize the knowledge you have gained during your experience. It can also be very helpful later on when studying for the RDN exam.

Anatomy of an Internship

DI rotations will take place in clinical care (also known as medical nutrition therapy, or MNT), food systems management, and community nutrition specialties. Each emphasis is further segmented into short-term experiences, or rotations, of supervised practice ranging from one week to multiple months, depending on the structure of the internship. All internships offer planned staff experience, and some offer an elective option—both will be defined later in the chapter. Next, we'll take a deep dive into the three main areas of dietetics practice.

Clinical Care / Medical Nutrition Therapy

The MNT experience is designed to give you broad-based, in-depth training in clinical care. In addition to a general nutrition therapy rotation, you may rotate through specialty areas, such as kidney disease, diabetes, cardiovascular disease, surgery, trauma/burns, oncology, or long-term care and rehabilitation. Ideally, you will work with a range of ages, from pediatrics to geriatrics. You will also gain experience in nutrition support, provided as both enteral and parenteral nutrition.

At the start of your clinical rotations, the majority of your time will be spent shadowing a preceptor or preceptors and learning how to function as a professional. As you progress in the program, you will be given greater responsibility, taking on patient assignments and more difficult learning experiences. Toward the end, you will be expected to assume the full responsibilities of a clinical dietitian, called planned staff experience, and function as an independent RDN. Of course, you'll still have access to other RDN preceptors who can assist you if the need arises, but, overall, this experience provides perspective on what it would be like to work solo, fosters self-confidence in basic skills, and promotes professionalism in the field.

Take this as an opportunity to prove to yourself and others that you are capable of running your own show! Also, keep in mind that planned staff experience can be in any area of practice, including the other specialties covered next, which allows you to pursue interests outside of clinical practice.

Food Systems Management

Food systems management encompasses a range of experiences, including food production and service, management, and administration. In this specialty, you will learn firsthand how RDNs can function in foodservice, retail and other food systems, management, and administrative areas of dietetics. Some programs may focus more on business management than the foodservice portion, or vice versa, but it's best to gain both experiences if possible.

In this part of your internship, you can and should work with individuals at all levels of food production, from the purchasing manager (also called procurement), to the frontline supervisors who manage the tray-line staff, to the executive chef and/or production manager who coordinates food preparation, as well as other professionals. You will learn how to coordinate and manage a foodservice operation safely, efficiently, and economically and how to manage people, payroll, and scheduling as well as conflicts and negotiations. To further bolster your business savvy, certain programs also have you develop a business plan either independently or in teams with the other interns and function in other, non-foodservice management roles.

Community and Public Health

In this final area, principles of nutrition are applied to groups of people or communities, typically through the implementation and evaluation of health-related programs. Rotations will take place with different community programs and agencies, depending on the internship location, and among diverse, often underserved populations. Options include local health departments, food banks, cooperative extension initiatives, and nutrition and food assistance programs for the elderly (such as Meals on Wheels) or for low-income families, such as the Special Supplemental Nutrition Program for Women, Infants, and Children (WIC) or Head Start.

At these community sites, you might counsel individuals or groups of clients to encourage healthful eating and lifestyle habits, or you might teach classes on nutrition topics, such as prenatal nutrition; diabetes or cardiovascular disease; meal planning on a budget; and tips for feeding infants, toddlers, and children—just to name a few! Other responsibilities might be evaluating grants, creating nutrition education materials, or leading supermarket or farmers market tours. We mentioned earlier that school nutrition programs have become a top priority in federal and state legislation, which has led to greater involvement from food and nutrition experts, including registered dietitians, in program development, implementation, and evaluation and improvement. As a dietetic intern, you may have the opportunity to work with a school nutrition dietitian on menu planning, recipe development, or nutrition education and outreach programs for students.

Make the Most of Every Rotation

The summary we've provided is only an overview of the kinds of activities you might encounter throughout your internship. Internships vary and so will the organizations you work with. It's a smart idea to ask for advice about the possible projects, goals, and objectives

SPECIAL INTEREST OR ELECTIVE ROTATIONS

Many internships offer students the opportunity to coordinate their own special interest rotations, or electives, which can last from 1 to 6 weeks. The experience depends on the intern's career goals and interest. This is the time to go for something you haven't yet learned in the internship or to build on and bolster your experiences in an additional area of practice you're interested in. Your program director will help you set up and/or approve your special intrest rotations. He or she will also be able to provide examples of elective rotations completed by previous dietetic interns.

you can set for yourself in each rotation. You should also tap into resources from your program director and each individual preceptor for their guidance and advice, both short-term during the internship and long-term over your career.

Distance Education and Internet Education

Distance programs originated to provide experiences in geographic areas where no formal DI or coordinated program was available. These programs may be right for you if your family or job responsibilities keep you in an area that may not have a DI or coordinated program in dietetics. Distance education programs often start with an initial one-week, on-campus orientation. Lodging and transportation during this time may or may not be the intern's responsibility. The remainder of the program—that is, instruction and course work, projects and assignments, and advisement—is administered electronically.

When it comes to supervised practice, in general, the distance education intern will need to coordinate much more of his or her own internship experience, which can be challenging. Preceptors and facilities will be subject to approval by the DI director and will require having appropriate contracts in place (if they aren't already). You and your program director will also need to make sure that you receive the right range of experiences and meet all required competencies, introduced earlier in the chapter. The benefit of distance learning is that you will be networking with colleagues and organizations in your own area. If this is an option you are considering, be sure to contact programs, speak with the program director and with current and former interns, and learn the logistics, challenges, and type of support the program offers.

Sample Dietetic Internships from Across the Country

To help you get a feel for some of the DI options, several accredited programs offered in the United States are highlighted here. Just remember, these are only a few examples among many more accredited programs. The ACEND website has a full list of DI programs with accreditation status.[2] (Note: Please refer to individual program websites for the most up-to-date information.)

Dietetic Internship-Only Programs

Arizona State University

The program's mission is to develop dietitians who have the skills necessary to transfer nutrition knowledge into application and high-quality entry-level practice. The program provides a strong core of dietetic experiences in which the interns will use knowledge gained in their undergraduate studies and graduate research to benefit the nutrition knowledge, health, and wellness of individuals and the community.

- **Annual enrollment:** 6
- **Program length:** 9 months
- **Emphasis:** research, wellness
- **Website:** https://snhp.asu.edu/programs/internships/dietetic-internship

California State University Fresno

This is a nine-month program with a culturally competent health promotion/disease prevention concentration. Its mission is to unlock the potential of future registered dietitian nutritionists through innovative and diverse postgraduate practice application while uniquely nourishing cultural competency in a variety of dietetic settings within Fresno County, the Fresno metropolitan area, and the Central San Joaquin Valley.

- **Annual enrollment:** 10
- **Program length:** 10 months
- **Emphasis:** culturally competent health promotion and disease prevention
- **Financial stipend for full-time nondegree:** $1,200
- **Website:** www.fresnostate.edu/jcast/fsn/degrees-programs/dieteticinternship/programoverview.html

Mayo Clinic/School of Health Sciences

There are two DI programs affiliated with the Mayo Clinic: a program located at the Mayo School of Health Sciences in Rochester, MN, and a program at the Mayo Clinic in Jacksonville, FL. Their emphases are in medical nutrition therapy and clinical nutrition, respectively. Both programs provide extensive patient interaction and clinical knowledge and skills, enabling graduates to deliver complete nutrition services in a variety of settings.

- **Annual enrollment:** 8 (MN); 9 (FL)
- **Program length:** 11 months (MN); 8 months (FL)
- **Emphasis:** nutrition therapy (MN); clinical nutrition (FL)
- **Website:** www.mayo.edu/mshs/careers/dietetics/dietetics -internship-minnesota and www.mayo.edu/mshs/careers /dietetics/dietetics-internship-florida

Montclair State University Dietetic Internship

This internship program consists of supervised practice as well as classroom education and the completion of six graduate credits. Interns rotate through various facilities to gain diverse experiences in the program's emphasis of nutrition therapy. Inpatient clinical rotations include medicine and surgery, intensive care, pediatrics, and long-term care; outpatient rotations provide experiences in diabetes, dialysis, and maternal nutrition. Additional rotations include school foodservice management, community nutrition programs (such as Head Start), cooperative extension, wellness programs, and research.

- **Annual enrollment:** 12
- **Program length:** 10 months
- **Emphasis:** MNT
- **Website:** www.montclair.edu/cehs/academics/departments /hns/academic-programs/dietetic-intern/

Sodexo Dietetic Internship

This internship is committed to providing high-quality supervised training for qualified graduates of an accredited didactic curriculum in dietetics. It offers full- and part-time training, promoting individualized educational experiences in a flexible manner to meet the unique needs of diverse dietetic interns. This DI also offers the option of distance education, which may include an online master's degree program through the University of Rhode Island while completing the supervised practice experiences. The Sodexo DI provides clinical, managerial, and community dietetics training.

- **Annual enrollment:** varies by campus (5 total in Massachusetts, New York, Pennsylvania, and Maryland/Washington, DC)
- **Program length:** varies by campus and program type
- **Emphasis:** leadership, MNT, diabetes, pediatric, weight management, senior living, wellness, or culinary
- **Estimated total tuition:** varies by campus
- **Website:** www.dieteticintern.com

University of North Carolina Greensboro

The mission of this DI program is to prepare competent, entry-level dietitians for positions in clinical, foodservice, and community nutrition to better serve individuals and their families, particularly in North Carolina. It features 10 weeks of preparation course work and 27 weeks of supervised practice plus a professional and community engagement project with a designated community partner. Affiliated supervised practice sites are located throughout North Carolina.

- **Annual enrollment:** 21
- **Program length:** 10 months
- **Emphasis:** professional and community engagement
- **Website:** http://hhs.uncg.edu/wordpress/ntr/dietetic -internship/

Virginia Polytechnic Institute and State University (Virginia Tech)

The program has two locations in Northern Virginia (Falls Church) and Blacksburg, providing interns the shared resources of both a large research-based university and the urban Washington, DC, area.

The program also provides interns with a variety and depth of experiences needed to work in many different professional practice settings. Its unique emphasis on leadership and professional development builds on interns' previous leadership positions and enables graduates to enter the profession ready to influence their workplace, their profession, and food and nutrition policy.

- **Annual enrollment:** 16
- **Program length:** 10 months
- **Emphasis:** leadership and professional development
- **Website:** www.hnfe.vt.edu/internship-nutrition_and _dietetics/index.html

The Pennsylvania State University Dietetic Internship

This program is committed to providing a broad range of experiences in order for future dietetics professionals to become familiar with the breadth of available opportunities. It emphasizes critical thinking skills and evidence-based learning while exploring many areas in the field of dietetics and prepares professionals for lifelong learning.

- **Annual enrollment:** 10
- **Program length:** 11 months
- **Emphasis:** leadership in diverse practice
- **Website:** http://nutrition.hhdev.psu.edu/internship/index.html

Missouri State

Offered by the biomedical sciences department, the DI at Missouri State prepares competent dietitian practitioners who are citizen scholars with expertise in either public affairs or rural health (the two concentration options). Interns receive training in practicums with health clinics, hospitals, public school systems, and community organizations, preparing them for a variety of dietetic career pathways. Missouri State also offers international experiences where interns can complete supervised rotations in another country for one week or a whole semester.

- **Annual enrollment:** 12
- **Program length:** 9 months

- **Emphasis:** public affairs, rural health
- **Website:** www.missouristate.edu/dietetics/graduate

Dietetic Internships Combined with a Graduate Program

US Military–Baylor Graduate Program in Nutrition

The Army DI was expanded in 2006 to be a combined master's degree/internship program. In this way, it's a two-phase, degree-producing program comprising the master's program in nutrition as well as the DI. The Phase 1 didactic portion is approximately nine months long and is completed at the Army Medical Department Center and Fort Sam Houston. The Phase 2 internship and research portion is 12 months long and is completed at one of three medical centers in Texas.

- **Annual enrollment:** 10
- **Program length:** 20 months
- **Emphasis:** military skills
- **Financial stipend for full-time degree:** $54,000
- **Website:** www.baylor.edu/graduate/nutrition/index .php?id=67970

University of Texas Health, School of Public Health

This is one of only a few combined master of public health–registered dietitian/DI programs in the United States. Its mission is to advance health and healthful living for children and families through innovative research; cutting-edge, community-based programs; and the dissemination of evidence-based practices. Dietetic interns learn through didactic work, supervised practice, and their final specialty practice rotation with staff experience in an area of public health nutrition selected by the intern.

- **Annual enrollment:** 9
- **Program length:** 22–24 months
- **Emphasis:** public health nutrition
- **Website:** https://sph.uth.edu/research/centers/dell /dietetic-internship-program

Loyola University Chicago

The mission of the Loyola University Chicago DI is to provide students with quality supervised practice within the context of a Jesuit, Catholic University. It offers two tracks: DI-only for 13 months or combined master of science/DI for 22 months. In both options, students benefit from the Marcella Niehoff School of Nursing's constructive and supportive environment, learning the leadership, communication, and management skills they need to pass the registration exam and enter dietetics practice.

- **Annual enrollment:** 20 (10 for each track)
- **Program length:** 22 months (graduate degree track); 13 months (nondegree)
- **Emphasis:** public health nutrition
- **Website:** www.luc.edu/nursing/dietetic_internships/

The University of Georgia

The DI is completed as part of a master's degree in foods and nutrition science. The internship component is completed during two consecutive summers, with additional course work during the academic year, through a wide variety of supervised practice sites in the Athens and Atlanta areas. The internship's mission is to prepare interns for a successful career in dietetics and encourage them to assume a leadership role in the profession and in society.

- **Annual enrollment:** 6
- **Program length:** 25 months
- **Emphasis:** community intervention and research, MNT
- **Financial stipend for full-time degree:** $22,596
- **Website:** www.fcs.uga.edu/fdn/graduate/dietetics.html

Programs in Candidacy for Accreditation

Candidacy for accreditation is a designation for programs that have not yet been fully accredited but have had at least one site visit and are being implemented according to the ACEND Accreditation Standards.[3] Graduates of a program with candidate for accreditation status are eligible, upon satisfactory completion of the program, to sit for the RDN credentialing exam. The following are two examples of new programs. Always check the ACEND website for the most up-to-date information on any new and upcoming programs.

Children's Hospital Colorado Dietetic Internship

The Children's Hospital Colorado DI is a newly developed program with this designation. It offers training in two concentrations: pediatrics and adult acute care. Its mission is to provide dietetic interns exceptional training to best prepare them for entry-level positions and to become leaders in clinical nutrition, nutrition education, and research for children, adults, and families.

- **Annual enrollment:** 6
- **Program length:** 10 months
- **Emphasis:** adult acute care, pediatrics
- **Website:** www.childrenscolorado.org/departments/nutrition /dietetic-internship-program

Wellness Workdays

Another candidate for accreditation that offers a unique distance education program, this internship is designed to meet the individual needs of prospective RDNs with a focus on worksite wellness and health promotion. With both full-time and part-time options, this internship has great flexibility depending on the intern's needs and can be completed at practice sites and with preceptors in the intern's local setting.

- **Annual enrollment:** 16 (full-time); 4 (part-time)
- **Program length:** 8 months (full-time); 11 months (part-time)
- **Emphasis:** worksite wellness and health promotion
- **Website:** www.wellnessworkdays.com/#/di/4570381141

Financial Aid Considerations

Being accepted into a DI program is a great accomplishment. Everything has a cost; how you plan to pay for this next step in your career is something to consider early on. Unless you enroll in a US military DI program, which offers excellent compensation and benefits, or a few other programs that offer stipend support, most internships involve tuition and fees. Just as you considered cost and financial support in your undergraduate program, it's important to consider financial support resources to help you finance the DI as well as other necessities, like health insurance (if applicable).

You may also need to cover housing, utilities, transportation, food, books and supplies, and other recommended materials for the internship, including a computer, diet analysis software, dietetic manuals, a calculator, binders, and so forth. Some programs may also require that you purchase a liability insurance policy. Our philosophy on this matter is simple: Get the best your money can buy while sticking to your budget.

Sources of Financial Aid

First, know that it is very unlikely (and highly discouraged) that you'll have the time to work during your internship. Therefore, other sources for funding your DI will need to be considered, most likely through scholarships and loans. Speak with your college program adviser and director about some of these possibilities. The Academy of Nutrition and Dietetics Foundation, for example, raises millions of dollars to support dietetics education, including internships, through scholarships. These are awarded competitively and are a great opportunity for dietetics students.

Financial aid or another loan program may be available through your program. This should be an important consideration when ranking programs during computer matching. Detailed information about federal grants and loans administered by the US Department of Education is available online (www.StudentAid.ed.gov). Additional sources include state higher education agencies and civic, professional, and community organizations or foundations. The financial aid office at your program's institution can also provide information about scholarship programs and private loan options.

If you seek financial aid, you can apply online by completing the Free Application for Federal Student Aid (FAFSA) and submitting it directly to the US Department of Education. Visit the FAFSA website (www.fafsa.ed.gov) for more information.

References

1. Accreditation Council for Education in Nutrition and Dietetics. *ACEND Accreditation Standards for Internship Programs in Nutrition & Dietetics Leading to the RD Credential.* http://www .eatrightacend.org/WorkArea/linkit.aspx?LinkIdentifier=id&ItemID =6442485379&libID=6442485357. Updated March 31, 2015. Accessed January 12, 2016.

2. Accreditation Council for Education in Nutrition and Dietetics. Dietetic internships. http://www.eatrightacend.org/ACEND/content .aspx?id=6442485424. Accessed January 12, 2016.

CHAPTER 5

The Registration Examination for Dietitians

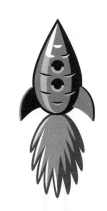

....

THOUGHT QUESTIONS

- Review the full Registration Examination for Dietitians Study Outline. What areas do you think you might be stronger in than others? Explain why—this is an important practice because it can help guide your dietetics education and supervised practice preparation.

- We've named a few resources for exam preparation. Search online for additional resources that you might consider. (We know they are out there!) Describe their format and approach to exam preparation.

- Do you know what type of learner you are? Take the online Index of Learning Styles (ILS) survey developed at North Carolina State University, which can help you identify if you are a sensing and intuitive, a visual and verbal, or a sequential and global learner. The survey can be found on the university website (www.engr.ncsu.edu/learning-styles

....

THE DAY WILL COME WHEN YOU'RE ELIGIBLE TO SIT FOR the Registration Examination for Dietitians. When it does, celebrate everything you've already accomplished, including years of course work and many hours of supervised practice. Successful completion of the examination means that you will be recognized as a registered dietitian nutritionist (RDN). Remember that the RDN credential is interchangeable with registered dietitian (RD). The aim of this chapter is to provide information, guidance, and tips for helping you feel confident about this next step and ensuring that you choose the right resources to successfully prepare for the exam.

RDN Exam 101

The Commission on Dietetic Registration (CDR), not to be confused with the Accreditation Council for Nutrition and Dietetics (ACEND), is the independent credentialing agency that awards the RDN (or RD) credential to qualified candidates. According to its mission statement, CDR "administers rigorous, valid and reliable credentialing processes to protect the public and meet the needs of nutrition and dietetics practitioners, employers and consumers."[1] All CDR certification programs are fully accredited by the National Commission for Certifying Agencies (NCCA), the accrediting arm of the Institute for Credentialing Excellence.

In order to award credentials, CDR contracts with Pearson VUE, an examination testing agency, to administer the registration exam. Through a certification testing program, the registration exam content is designed to evaluate a potential candidate's readiness to practice at the entry level. You'll be tested on a range of dietetic concepts, procedures, and logic. You'll need to decipher graphs, tables, and formulas; solve nutritional problems; and make management decisions.

It is also important to know that the exam is administered as a computer-based test and, more specifically, as computer adaptive testing (CAT).[2] This is a type of electronic testing that administers questions strategically and efficiently in order to determine the test taker's competence. CAT is typically shorter than traditional pen-and-paper tests and provides you with a score immediately upon

EXAM RESOURCES: FROM THE COMMITTEE ON DIETETIC REGISTRATION

- *Registration Examination for Dietitians Handbook for Candidates*
- *Registration Examination for Dietitians Study Outline*, which is up-dated every five years to reflect measured changes in practice identified in the entry-level dietetics practice audit

Both are available at the CDR's website under the "Graduating Student Information" section (www.cdrnet.org/program-director /grad-info-student).

completion. More specifics and answers to common questions about the computer test will be provided later in the chapter.

Application for Eligibility

Before taking the registration exam, you must apply to become eligible. To start this process, your dietetic internship, coordinated program, or individualized supervised practice pathway (ISPP) program director will fill out an online form to notify CDR that you are eligible to take the test. When CDR has processed the information and your eligibility has been established, the testing agency (Pearson VUE) will be contacted. Pearson will then send the candidate an "Authorization to Test" e-mail, a link to the *Registration Examination for Dietitians Handbook for Candidates*, and instructions for submitting the application fee, which is currently $200 for the registration examination. The entire process, from when your director notifies CDR to when you are contacted by Pearson VUE, typically takes three to four weeks.

Next, when registering for your examination on Pearson VUE's website, you will need to do the following:

- Sign in to the CDR/Pearson VUE web portal using the username and password you received upon creating your Pearson VUE account.
- Begin the scheduling process by choosing your exam under the "Pre-approved Exams" section of the website.

- Select, on the "Additional Questions from CDR" page, whether or not your name should be released along with your exam scores to your program director.
- Agree not to disclose any information about the exam to anyone else. In order to proceed with the application, you must select "I Agree."
- Use the calendar tool to see available test times and select a date.
- Review the appointment details and proceed to checkout to pay for the testing appointment.
- Agree to the CDR policies to schedule your exam. The system will display the exam policies for cancellation and rescheduling.

If online registration is completed successfully, you will receive another e-mail from Pearson VUE to confirm your examination time and location. You have one year from the time you are authorized by CDR to schedule and take your examination. If you do not take the exam during this one-year period or if you do not pass the exam, you must contact CDR to be reauthorized to retake the test. You will also have to repay the examination fee and wait 45 calendar days between testing experiences. For other questions about special accommodations due to a disability and required documentation for accommodations, refer to CDR's *Registration Examination for Dietitians Handbook for Candidates*.[3] All accommodation requests must be submitted to Pearson VUE using the forms found on their website.

Anatomy of the Exam

All examinees are given a minimum of 125 questions including 25 pretest questions (which will not be scored). These pretest questions are being tested for future exams, but you won't know which questions they are, so concentrate on answering all the questions as best as you can. Although you must answer at least 125 questions to receive a score, the maximum number of questions is 145. This range allows you more questions to answer correctly, if needed, to demonstrate your competency. See Figure 5.1.

FIGURE 5.1.

Flow chart of registration eligibility application processing

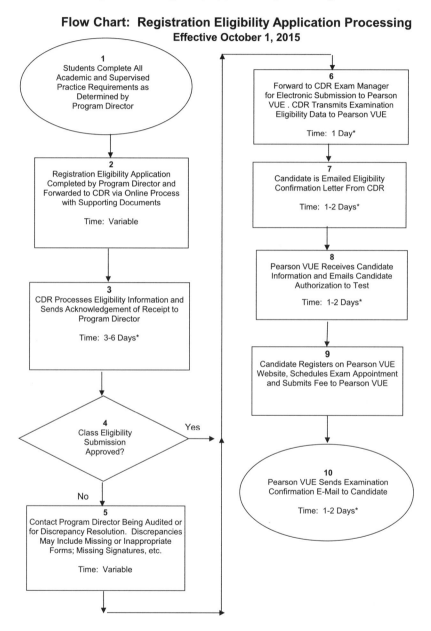

Flow Chart: Registration Eligibility Application Processing
Effective October 1, 2015

1
Students Complete All Academic and Supervised Practice Requirements as Determined by Program Director

2
Registration Eligibility Application Completed by Program Director and Forwarded to CDR via Online Process with Supporting Documents

Time: Variable

3
CDR Processes Eligibility Information and Sends Acknowledgement of Receipt to Program Director

Time: 3-6 Days*

4
Class Eligibility Submission Approved?

Yes

No

5
Contact Program Director Being Audited or for Discrepancy Resolution. Discrepancies May Include Missing or Inappropriate Forms; Missing Signatures, etc.

Time: Variable

6
Forward to CDR Exam Manager for Electronic Submission to Pearson VUE . CDR Transmits Examination Eligibility Data to Pearson VUE

Time: 1 Day*

7
Candidate is Emailed Eligibility Confirmation Letter From CDR

Time: 1-2 Days*

8
Pearson VUE Receives Candidate Information and Emails Candidate Authorization to Test

Time: 1-2 Days*

9
Candidate Registers on Pearson VUE Website, Schedules Exam Appointment and Submits Fee to Pearson VUE

10
Pearson VUE Sends Examination Confirmation E-Mail to Candidate

Time: 1-2 Days*

* Business Days

Source: Commission on Dietetic Registration

HOW IT WORKS: COMPUTER-BASED TESTS

The registration exam is a computer-based, multiple-choice test. If you've taken the GREs, you will be familiar with the testing environment and question procedure. Here are the rules:

- The exam appointment is for 3 hours, which includes 2½ hours to take the examination and 30 minutes to complete an introductory tutorial and exit questionnaire.

- This tutorial provides instructions on taking the examination and a set of practice questions. A practice test is included in the *Study Guide for the Registration Examination for Dietitians*. Exam candidates can purchase the guide through the Academy of Nutrition and Dietetics store (www.eatrightstore.org).

- There is no skipping of questions to ponder and return later. You must answer each question as it comes before the computer will offer the next question.

- Items are administered in random order according to test specifications.

There are four domains, each with multiple subtopics that you'll be asked about on the exam (see Figure 5.2). These domains reflect competencies and knowledge that you should have gained during the didactic dietetic program and supervised practice preparation. They are updated regularly based on measured dietetics practice. The most recent dietetics practice audit took place in 2015, and based on this report, a new exam outline will take effect January 1, 2017.[4] Therefore, make sure to use the most up-to-date version of the CDR's Registration Examination for Dietitians Study Outline, *Handbook for Candidates*, and other materials.

Tips and Resources for Exam Preparation

In the weeks and days leading up to the exam, it is very common to feel stressed and to doubt your knowledge. Although it is easier said than done, you will stay more focused and better prepared for the exam by figuring out ways to cope with these feelings, like utilizing wellness and counseling services or making time for physical activity

FIGURE 5.2.
Domain areas of the credentialing examination

DOMAIN I: Principles of Dietetics (12%)	DOMAIN II: Nutrition Care for Individuals and Groups (50%)	DOMAIN III: Management of Food and Nutrition Programs and Services (21%)	DOMAIN IV: Foodservice Systems (17%)
Topic A: Food Science and Nutrient Composition of Foods	Topic A: Screening and Assessment	Topic A: Functions of Management	Topic A: Menu Development
Topic B: Nutrition and Supporting Science	Topic B: Diagnosis	Topic B: Human Resources	Topic B: Procurement, Production, Distribution, and Service
Topic C: Education and Communication	Topic C: Planning and Intervention	Topic C: Financial Management	Topic C: Sanitation and Safety
Topic D: Research	Topic D: Monitoring and Evaluation	Topic D: Marketing and Public Relations	Topic D: Equipment and Facility Planning
Topic E: Management Concepts		Topic E: Quality Improvement	Topic E: Sustainability

or relaxing activities such as yoga or cooking—whatever works for you from previous experience.

Solid preparation leading up to test day also helps relieve some of the potential anxiety. After all of the academic classes and supervised practice hours you've completed, a month of exam preparation is usually sufficient. Do not wait too long! We recommend taking the

WANT TO PRACTICE FOR THE EXAM?

Many test prep books and review courses are available. To find resources or exam study materials, ask your advisers or mentors for recommendations; also ask your peers and recently registered dietitians to hear their experiences. The Academy of Nutrition and Dietetics offers an online student exam prep (StEP) resource, with a database of more than 700 questions on topics such as basic dietetics principles, nutrition care, management, and foodservice systems, plus practice quizzes and test-taking tips from successful RDNs. The resource is available for purchase at the eatrightSTORE (www.eatrightstore.org).

test as soon as you can after completing your course work or supervised practice while allowing yourself at least a few weeks to review exam material. After you've picked a date, set up a study calendar to stay on track and schedule time to cover everything you need. You may also consider a review course, which can reduce some of the work involved in preparing for the registration exam because it offers structured lectures, study materials, sample questions, and plenty of practice. Although they can be expensive, review courses are usually designed to help focus your attention on the material that matters most.

Test Day

The evening before the exam, prepare everything you need to take with you the next day. It is imperative that you take your valid government-issued photo ID. Without the ID, you will not be admitted to the exam. Get a good night's sleep, eat a well-balanced breakfast the morning of the exam, and allow yourself plenty of time to travel to your testing center.

Once seated at the testing station, you'll have a 30-minute tutorial to become familiar with the computer process and to review the instructions. An online or simple handheld calculator will be provided for you by the testing center, so get familiar with this before starting. You have exactly 2½ hours to complete the exam, which begins when you click on your first question. Remember that after advancing you cannot go back to review answers, change responses, or skip questions, so give each question adequate consideration before moving on. If you need to leave the room in the middle of the exam, you must have the proctor's permission, and you will not get that time back (you cannot pause or extend the testing time).

Fortunately, you'll get your results right at the testing center, following completion of the exam. A score of 25 or higher (on a scale of 1 to 50) is needed to pass.

If You Don't Pass...

SITUATIONS THAT CANCEL YOUR RIGHT TO TAKE THE EXAM

- It's been over a year since the date listed on your authorization to test e-mail.
- You fail to cancel your testing appointment before the 48-hour/two-day deadline.
- On test day, you arrive late or don't have a valid government-issued photo ID, or the name on your valid government-issued ID does not match the name on your Pearson VUE profile.
- You are caught cheating.
- You sit for the exam but fail to complete it within 2½ hours.
- You abort the examination before it's completed.

There is always a second chance if you don't pass the exam on your first try, and this doesn't mean you won't be a successful RDN. If you complete the exam but do not get a passing score, you can apply for reauthorization to retake the exam by contacting CDR directly to reapply and pay another examination fee to Pearson VUE. And remember that even though the RDN credential may be necessary for certain careers, a degree in nutrition and dietetics alone still offers viable career options. Some examples are certain jobs in food sales, public health nutrition, and foodservice management. Someone with a degree in dietetics, nutrition, or food science could certainly be a step ahead of someone who does not have this type of education.

References

1.   Commission on Dietetic Registration. About CDR. https://www.cdrnet.org/about. Accessed January 12, 2016.

2.   Commission on Dietetic Registration. Entry-level Registration Examinations for Dietitians and Dietetic Technicians Q&A / fact sheet. https://www.cdrnet.org/vault/2459/web/files/CBTFACT2014.pdf. Published September 2014. Accessed January 12, 2016.

3.   Commission on Dietetic Registration. Registration Examination for Dietitians Handbook for Candidates. https://www.cdrnet.org/vault/2459/web/files/CDRRDHandbook2015-1.pdf. Accessed January 12, 2016.

4.   Commission on Dietetic Registration. 2015 dietetics practice audit. https://www.cdrnet.org/2015-dietetics-practice-audit. Accessed January 12, 2016.

CHAPTER 6

Secrets to Success: An Orientation for the New RDN

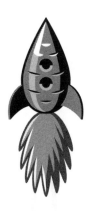

THOUGHT QUESTIONS

- Join the Academy of Nutrition and Dietetics. Name three to five benefits of being an Academy member that appeal to you.

- Based on the full list of dietetic practice groups (DPGs) listed on the Academy's eatrightPRO website (www.eatright pro.org/resources/membership/academy-groups/dietetic -practice-groups), name the top three groups that you would join, and explain why. Do any of these offer special opportunities for members?

- Sign up for the Academy's *Daily News* e-mail and monitor for a full week. Did you learn anything from the news and research updates? Name a few topics that appealed to you most and describe what you learned.

C ONGRATULATIONS AND WELCOME TO THE WORLD OF being a registered dietitian nutritionist (RDN)! You've worked hard in your education and training for this gold-standard credential in food and nutrition, and now the public can be assured of your expertise. In this chapter, we'll show you ways to reach your full potential in dietetics—from engaging with your professional organization, to advocating in the public policy arena, to giving back to your community through volunteering, to obtaining specialized certifications in certain dietetics practice areas. We'll walk you through the continuing professional education (CPE) requirements involved with maintaining the RDN (also called registered dietitian [RD]) credential. We'll also delve into the importance of and opportunities for mentorship in dietetics. Even if you have not yet taken and passed the registration exam, it's never too early to read ahead and preview some of the responsibilities you have as an RDN.

Maintaining Your Credential: Continuing Professional Education

To maintain the RDN credential, you must earn 75 hours of CPE credits during each five-year period. The Commission on Dietetic Registration (CDR), which you'll remember also administers the exam and awards the credentials, is responsible for monitoring continuing education and ensuring that you not only maintain the knowledge and skills to continue practicing as a dietitian but also develop professionally in your own career path. Remember that the RDN or RD credentials are interchangeable, legally protected titles. Only dietetics professionals who have completed the requirements outlined in previous chapters can call themselves an RDN—credentials that represent competence to provide services to patients and clients.

Staying up-to-date on developments in food and nutrition science is more than a requirement for your credential—it also builds your knowledge, enhances your skills, and will help advance your career. We believe that learning should never cease, especially in nutrition and dietetics—a relatively young and dynamic science that is continuously evolving with advancements in technology and research. CPE helps you stay abreast of these developments and proves your competence to practice.

Essential Practice Competencies

Starting in June 2015, the Essential Practice Competencies for the Commission on Dietetic Registration's Credentialed Nutrition and Dietetics Practitioners were implemented, which now provide validated standards for the RDN credential.[1] Building on the entry-level competencies described in the previous chapter, the essential practice competencies "define the knowledge, skills, judgment, and attitude requirements throughout a practitioner's career, across practice, and within focus areas."[2] In that way, the purpose of practice competencies is to guide continuing education and professional development, advance an individual's practice, and define the area of focus or expertise.

There are 14 essential practice competencies, composed of 9 core competencies and 5 functional competencies. Within each essential practice competency, also referred to as a sphere, there are varying practice competencies, which describe the identifiable components of expected performance, including the knowledge, skills, judgment, and attitudes needed for both general practice and a particular practice focus.[3] They were developed to be (1) broad enough to encompass the range of specialties and unique roles within the dietetics profession; (2) descriptive of the different practice roles between the RDN and nutrition and dietetics technician, registered (NDTR) credentials; and (3) applicable to all credentialed nutrition practitioners.

Background on the Professional Development Portfolio

Prior to the new essential practice competencies, RDNs completed continuing professional education to align with a professional development portfolio (PDP), based on knowledge-based learning need codes. It is important to know, because PDP is still a relevant and utilized term, referring to the umbrella process that includes planning and logging your professional development (regardless of the switch to essential practice competencies).

In short, the PDP is a personalized learning plan that you design on your own, with the goal of advancing your career and knowledge as a registered dietitian.[4] RDNs identify their own learning needs or interests and then create and execute a plan based on this assessment. The shift to a PDP for continuing education was based on research suggesting that optimal outcomes occur when "each practitioner identifies knowledge and skills needed for professional competence, uses appropriate educational methods, and develops individualized strategies to implement what has been learned by applying it to professional practice."[5] Although CDR has transitioned to using an essential practice competencies program, RDNs will continue to follow their current PDP until their next recertification cycle, when they will develop a new learning plan using The Goal Wizard (explained next) that adopts the recent changes.

Developing a Learning Plan: The Goal Wizard

The process of developing your PDP has been condensed into three simple steps. In the previous system, RDNs would write their goals and learning plan. Now, a new program called The Goal Wizard has been developed to assist you with identifying the essential practice competency goals and performance indicators relevant to your practice as an RDN. It does this by asking you a series of questions and then applying a decision algorithm to make recommendations.[6] For a tutorial, visit the CDR website (www.cdrnet.org/competencies-for-practitioners), which provides additional resources to understand the new essential practice competencies.

This step covers professional self-reflection, learning needs assessment, and the learning plan development. The next steps are

- submitting and gaining approval for the learning plan from CDR,
- maintaining an activity log of earned CPE units, and
- conducting a professional development evaluation.

Together, this process will take place every five years, based on the date you first became registered. You may feel a little overwhelmed by this process, especially if you're a new graduate or are using the essential practice competencies for the first time. That's normal, and, fortunately, CDR offers a range of introductory materials to explain the process. You can also contact CDR staff directly with any questions.

Ways to Earn Continuing Professional Education Credits

There are a number of ways to earn the 75 CPE hours. One place to start is the "CPE Offerings and Resources" section of CDR's website, where there is a CPE database of all activities that have been preapproved by CDR for CPE units.[7] Professional conferences are one of the most popular ways of earning CPEs because they also offer an opportunity to network, in addition to participating in lectures, poster sessions, and other events that have been approved for CPEs. Conferences take place across a variety of specialties and practice areas.

TOP FOOD, NUTRITION, AND HEALTH CONFERENCES

- Food and Nutrition Conference and Exhibition (www.eatright.org/fnce)
- Clinical Nutrition Week (www.nutritioncare.org)
- International Congress of Dietetics (www.internationaldietetics.org/congress.aspx)
- National Restaurant Association Show (https://show.restaurant.org)
- State Dietetic Association Meetings (www.eatright.org/affiliates)
- DPG-sponsored conferences (see individual DPG websites)
- Experimental Biology (www.experimentalbiology.org)
- Society for the Study of Ingestive Behavior (www.ssib.org)

In addition to conferences, there are also CPE programs available online, such as audio lectures or webinars. You may read peer-reviewed journal articles, complete self-study activities, or attend case presentations to gain CPEs. Holding leadership positions in dietetics-related national, state, or district organizations, as well as completing academic course work or specialty certifications

FINANCIAL SUPPORT FOR CPE Although there are free CPE opportunities, others can come at a cost. The Academy's Foundation offers financial support to members who apply and qualify for support that can help offset the cost of continuing education. For example, the Karen Lechowich Continuing Education Award offers funds every year to a recent member of the Academy of Nutrition and Dietetics (a member of less than five years) to attend the annual Food and Nutrition Conference and Exhibition (FNCE). Your employer may also have opportunities for reimbursement for CPE

(discussed later in this chapter), can also qualify for CPEs. For a full list of potential activities, visit the "Center for Professional Development" section of the Academy of Nutrition and Dietetics—called "the Academy" by many in the field—website for online and in-person opportunities.[8]

Publications, such as the *Journal of the Academy of Nutrition and Dietetics*, *Today's Dietitian*, and state, dietetic practice group (DPG), or member interest group (MIG) newsletters, may also list CPE events. Another place that can keep you informed is the "Professional and Career Resources" section of the US Food and Nutrition Information Center.[9]

OTHER RECENT CONTINUING PROFESSIONAL EDUCATION UPDATES

CPE Unit Rollover: Although the goal is a minimum of 75 CPE units per five-year reporting period, you may earn many more than that. As of 2011, the CDR allows a 15-credit rollover, meaning you are allowed to carry over 15 credits completed within the last 75 days of the cycle, but only if you submit the PDP activity log on or by March 17 and your learning plan is submitted for the upcoming cycle within 120 days of completing the first activity you intend to log for CPE rollover.

Ethics CPE Activity: RDNs and NDTRs must complete a minimum of one CPE unit in ethics during each five-year recertification cycle.

DID YOU KNOW YOUR ACADEMY MEMBERSHIP CAN DO THAT?

Academy members have access to a number of resources. The Evidence Analysis Library (EAL; www.andeal.org) is an online library of nutritional research and evidence-based guidelines on important dietetics practice questions. Most of the publications are systematic reviews or evidence-based assessments of food and nutrition-related science on certain topics. These reviews are performed by expert Academy members based on predefined, objective, and transparent criteria. The goal is to evaluate, synthesize, and grade the strength of the evidence to support conclusions on important issues.

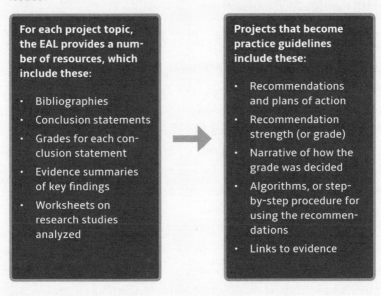

For each project topic, the EAL provides a number of resources, which include these:

- Bibliographies
- Conclusion statements
- Grades for each conclusion statement
- Evidence summaries of key findings
- Worksheets on research studies analyzed

Projects that become practice guidelines include these:

- Recommendations and plans of action
- Recommendation strength (or grade)
- Narrative of how the grade was decided
- Algorithms, or step-by-step procedure for using the recommendations
- Links to evidence

Your Professional Organization: Academy of Nutrition and Dietetics

Many would argue that without a professional governing organization, a profession cannot exist. As we introduced in Chapter 1, the Academy is the professional organization and governing body of the dietetics profession. It is the largest organization food and nutrition professionals, representing more than 75,000 individuals, from students to entry-level RDNs to experienced RDNs, as well as other dietetics practitioners holding undergraduate and advanced degrees in nutrition and dietetics. Its suborganizations by state or district affiliate, dietetics practice area, or special interest will be described in the next few sections. The Academy is committed to improving health and advancing the profession of dietetics through research, education, and advocacy. It offers intellectual stimulation, ongoing education, and leadership and networking opportunities for members while also protecting and promoting the profession. The Academy also acts as a unified voice for RDNs, advocating for representation and rights as a profession while also serving the public by optimizing health through food and nutrition.

Academy of Nutrition and Dietetics Groups

State Affiliates and District Affiliates

All 50 states, plus Puerto Rico, the District of Columbia, and the American Overseas Dietetic Association, are represented in the Academy. When you become a member, you are automatically part of your own state's affiliate group. However, you can be a member of another state association, for example, if you have just recently moved or if you live and work in different states.

Dietetic Practice Groups and Member Interest Groups

Because the Academy brings together diverse food and nutrition professionals from all facets of practice—NDTRs, foodservice administrators, chefs, clinical dietitians, community nutrition professionals, students, clinical researchers, educators, consultants, entrepreneurs, and more—members may also find it beneficial to network with others who have similar interests or are within a certain specialty. The DPGs and MIGs offer this opportunity. More information about specific Academy groups is available online.[10]

- DPGs are professional interest groups that enable members to enhance their specialized knowledge, share practice tips, and establish relationships with colleagues from all over the world. The types of DPGs range across many specialties, and because there's no limit to how many you can join, many practitioners belong to multiple groups.
- MIGs differ from DPGs by focusing on specific interests or commonalities outside the practice of dietetics. MIGs reflect the diversity of Academy members and the public we serve. A few examples include Thirty and Under in Nutrition and Dietetics, the National Organization of Men in Nutrition (founded by your authors, Kyle and Milton), Chinese Americans in Dietetics and Nutrition, and Latinos and Hispanics in Dietetics and Nutrition, to name a few.

What Are the Benefits of Academy Groups?

DPGs and MIGs host educational conferences and publish newsletters to inform members of developments in the field that could alter practice and improve delivery of services to clients. Members have an opportunity to get involved on the national and the local level by running for elected offices or serving on committees, contributing to Academy projects and legislative initiatives, authoring books or media publications, creating educational videos or handouts, and reviewing Academy position papers.

JOIN THE ACADEMY'S REFERRAL NETWORK

Academy members can choose to be listed in the "Find an Expert" directory, which is an online nutrition and dietetics referral service accessible to consumers. The directory may be helpful for those in a consulting business or private practice to raise awareness of their services. For information about how to join the referral service, send an e-mail to findnrd@eatright.org. Once you are listed, consumers and companies alike can search for your services by specialty and state using the online directory, located as a "Find an Expert" link on the Academy's consumer site (www.eatright.org).

All DPGs and MIGs require membership dues, paid upon renewal of your Academy membership. Keep in mind that these professional dues may be considered business-related expenses. Check with a tax professional to determine what can be used for a deduction.

Resources Available to Academy Members

For subscription and access information for the following printed and online publications, go to the Academy 's online Member Center (www.eatrightPRO.org).

- *Journal of the Academy of Nutrition and Dietetics*: This is the premier source for the practice and the science of food, nutrition, and dietetics.
- *Food & Nutrition Magazine*: The Academy's magazine covers nutrition, food, and health topics; practice tips; and resources for professional and personal growth.
- EatrightSTORE: All professional, client education, and consumer publications and other resources are available for purchase through the online store (www.eatrightstore.org). Academy members receive a discount on most products.
- ACEND Update: This resource communicates accreditation decisions and updates relating to processes and procedures in dietetics education.
- *Daily News*: The daily e-mail newsletter summarizes the latest news on food, nutrition, and health.
- *Eat Right Weekly*: The weekly newsletter covers updates in various practice areas: "On the Pulse of Public Policy," "CPE Corner," career resources, research briefs, member updates, philanthropy, awards, and grants.
- *Student Scoop*: The online newsletter is exclusively for dietetics students.
- *MNT Provider*: The monthly newsletter has resources for essential practice management, including nutrition practice guidelines and the complexities of coding, coverage, Medicare, and other reimbursement topics.

- *Kids Eat Right News Bite*: The quarterly newsletter highlights the great work to help children eat right around the world.

Other Nutrition Organizations

The Appendix lists several nutrition-related organizations that you may consult during your career as an RDN. Some of these also offer professional memberships. As you begin to find a niche, you may find value in joining complementary health-related organizations such as:

- American Association of Diabetes Educators (www.diabeteseducator.org)
- American Society for Nutrition (www.nutrition.org)
- American Society for Parenteral and Enteral Nutrition (www.nutritioncare.org)
- Association of Nutrition and Foodservice Professionals (www.anfponline.org)
- Institute of Food Technologists (www.ift.org)
- International Association of Culinary Professionals (www.iacp.com)
- National Restaurant Association (www.restaurant.org)
- Retail Dietitians Business Alliance (www.retaildietitians.com)
- School Nutrition Association (www.schoolnutrition.org)
- Society for Nutrition Education and Behavior (www.sneb.org)

Staying Current

As we mentioned earlier, when you transition from student to working RDN, staying current and connected to the field is not only necessary for continuing education but is also immensely valuable in making you the best professional you can be. It does take some work, but we have tips and strategies to make it easier for you!

- Subscribe to the Academy's *Daily News* e-mail newsletter (mentioned previously), which summarizes many current headlines influencing the profession and provides a roundup of the top research findings for the week as of each Friday.

- Take full advantage of the Academy's *Journal of the Academy of Nutrition and Dietetics*, a resource for peer-reviewed scientific research, reviews and position papers, and editorials or other articles for the profession. Take the time each month to browse the journal, and mark the articles that you plan to read more closely.

- Review abstracts of research from other journals as well, which can be found on the publishers' websites or via PubMed, the government's database for research publications. Abstracts offer only an overview of research. Use abstracts to help you identify studies of interest for a more thorough review of the complete article. In your monthly *Journal of the Academy of Nutrition and Dietetics*, there is an abstract and periodicals section that can help identify articles in various subject areas that you may find useful for keeping up on the science.

- Join professional listservs (e-mail subscriptions), such as that of your DPG(s), MIG(s), or state affiliate(s). Staying connected with colleagues will also help you keep up with what's going on in the professional world of food and nutrition.

- For more ideas, see the following resource lists, where we identify some of the top sources of nutrition information to get you started. These may or may not require paid subscription for full access. Remember, your employer might be able to cover the costs of resources for continuing education, so be sure to ask!

Specialist Certifications

After you have gained a few years of experience as an RDN—or if you already have an interest in advanced study—you may wish to pursue specialized practice areas. This requires extensive practice hours in the specialty and passing a comprehensive examination, but it may be necessary for the more prestigious positions. Certified specialists

FOOD, NUTRITION, AND HEALTH RESOURCES

Online Resources and Newsletters

Agriculture Research Service Food and Nutrition Research Briefs

American Heart Association's Resources for Professionals

Berkeley's Wellness Letter

Center for Science in the Public Interest

Daily News

Eat Right Weekly

Feeding Kids (www.nutrition forkids.com)

Food Marketing Institute (FMI)

FoodSafety.gov

Grocery Manufacturers Association (GMA)

Harvard Health Letters

International Food Information Council (FIC)

Maternal and Child Health (MCH) Research to Practice

National Food Service Management (NFSM) Institute's Insight

National Restaurant Association

Nutrition Action Health Letter

Nutrition Insights (USDA)

SmartBrief for Nutritionists

Student Scoop

The Johns Hopkins Medical Letter: Health After 50

Today's Dietitian magazine

Tufts University Health & Nutrition Letter

Peer-Reviewed Journals

American Journal of Clinical Nutrition

American Journal of Public Health

Appetite

Archives of Internal Medicine

British Medical Journal

Cambridge Scientific Abstracts

Circulation

Diabetes

Diabetes/Metabolism Research and Reviews

Family Economics and Nutrition Review

International Journal of Eating Disorders

International Journal of Obesity

Journal of the Academy of Nutrition and Dietetics

Journal of the American College of Nutrition

Journal of the American Medical Association

Journal of Nutrition

Journal of Nutrition Education and Behavior

Journal of Parenteral and Enteral Nutrition

New England Journal of Medicine

Nutrition in Clinical Practice

Nutrition: International Journal of Applied and Basic Nutritional Sciences

Obesity Research

Topics in Clinical Nutrition

also receive substantial CPE credits toward their professional development. Check with the board-certifying agency for specific requirements. CDR is also the credentialing agency for the following specialist board certifications, which recognize individuals for expertise in specialty areas:

- Board-certified specialist in gerontological nutrition (CSG)
- Board-certified specialist in oncology nutrition (CSO)
- Board-certified specialist in pediatric nutrition (CSP)
- Board-certified specialist in renal nutrition (CSR)
- Board-certified specialist in sports dietetics (CSSD)

If you'd like to learn more about these credentials, visit the CDR website (www.cdrnet.org/certifications/board-certified-specialist). Each specialist certification has specific requirements, so we encourage due diligence to determine if any are right for you.

Other continuing education opportunities are the CDR certificate of training programs in either adult or childhood and adolescent weight management. These comprehensive training programs were developed by registered dietitians, physicians, and other experts and include topics such as case management, nutrition assessment, environmental and genetic issues, prevention, physical activity, and behavioral management.

Mentors

It's never too early or too late in your dietetics career to find a great mentor. Having someone you can look to for guidance, coaching, and advice about the nutrition world is valuable for many reasons. You can bet he or she was in your shoes at one point, made many of the mistakes and learned from them, and moved on to other exciting challenges. A mentor might not have all the answers, but it helps to bounce ideas off of someone you trust. Balancing your decisions with the wisdom of experienced practitioners will serve you well.

Where Do You Find a Mentor?

A mentor can be anyone you relate to, whom you admire and respect, or whom you might aspire to be like in the future: educators and

ADDITIONAL CERTIFICATION PROGRAMS OF INTEREST TO RDNS

The following programs are certification programs that can qualify toward your CPE requirements. Check the CDR's *PDP Guide Appendix* for the most up-to-date list of approved certifications.

- Board certified—advanced diabetes management: American Association of Diabetes Educators and American Nurses Credentialing Center Commission on Certification (www.nursingworld.org/ANCC)
- Certified diabetes educator: National Certification Board for Diabetes Educators (www.ncbde.org)
- Certified nutrition support clinician: National Board of Nutrition Support Certification, Inc (www.nutritioncertify.org)
- NCSF-certified personal trainer: National Council on Strength and Fitness (www.ncsf.org)
- International board-certified lactation consultant: International Board of Lactation Consultant Examiners (www.iblce.org)
- ACE clinical exercise specialist, group fitness instructor, lifestyle and weight management coach consultant, or personal trainer: American Council on Exercise (www.acefitness.org)
- ACSM-certified personal trainer, health/fitness instructor or director, exercise specialist, or program director: American College of Sports Medicine (www.acsm.org)
- Certified in family and consumer sciences: American Association of Family and Consumer Sciences (www.aafcs.org)
- Certified health education specialist: National Commission for Health Education Credentialing (www.nchec.org)
- Certified professional in healthcare quality: Healthcare Quality Certification Commission, National Association for Healthcare Quality (www.nahq.org)
- Certified strength and conditioning specialist or NSCA-certified personal trainer: National Strength and Conditioning Association Certification Commission (www.nsca.org)
- Certified food scientist: Institute of Food Technologists (www.ift.org)
- NASM-certified personal trainer: National Academy of Sports Medicine (www.nasm.org)
- National certified counselor: National Board for Certified Counselors (www.nbcc.org)

A Closer Look

Mentors Pave the Way to Success

Before embarking on finding a mentor, define your goals. What do you want to achieve? Are you thinking of, or embarking on, a new career focus? Perhaps there is a specific area of focus you need to learn more about—business skills, Web development, social media, public speaking, advanced clinical skills, and so on. You also may know of a potential mentor whom you would like to approach about developing a mentor-mentee relationship. Perhaps it is someone you would like to model the next stage of your career after. Ask if he or she would be willing to mentor you. Because you will decide on the time commitment and focus together, you don't need to be concerned that it is "too much to ask." As someone once told me, "If you don't ask, the answer is already no." There's a good chance you will find yourself with a mentor you have admired and can learn a great deal from. Think about how you want to learn and develop, and take that next step!

Excerpt from Nutrition Entrepreneur's Ventures Newsletter, 2012. *Written by Elysa Jacobs Cruse, MS, RD, manager of corporate wellness for Pitney Bowes. Elysa was the Corporate Health Specialty Group chair for the Nutrition Entrepreneurs DPG for two years and continues to collaborate and benchmark with the group. Used with permission.*

employers, community members, local business owners, relatives, or close friends. As a member of the Academy, you can and should take advantage of all the DPGs and other networking groups that have mentor programs.

How Do You Establish the Relationship?

After finding a potential mentor, spend time together, perhaps on a committee or in a professional group, and learn more about the potential mentor. Once you feel comfortable, formally ask the person

Top 10 reasons to be mentored

It is a great way to...

10. find your niche in the nutrition world.

9. gather top-notch resources so you can set realistic and attainable goals.

8. get advice, direction, or encouragement from another RDN who has already traveled a similar path and can help you find your way to where you want to go.

7. fine-tune your decision-making skills to make your dream a reality. Live your vision!

6. get direction for common questions about the way you want to advance your career.

5. learn when it is time to consult a coach, accountant, attorney, etc.

4. learn how to stop procrastinating and be accountable for your progress and success.

3. determine your ideal job so that you can enjoy the work you are doing.

2. help you avoid common pitfalls in your career path so that you realize success.

1. help unlock your potential to become the RDN that you have always wanted to be.

Excerpt from Nutrition Entrepreneur's Ventures Newsletter, *2012. Written by Rebecca Bitzer, MS, RD, LD, CEDRD, president of Rebecca Bitzer & Associates, a nutrition counseling practice in Maryland. At the time of writing, she was on the Nutrition Entrepreneurs DPG Board as mentor coordinator and on the NE Board as private practice chair. Used with permission.*

if he or she will consider serving as your mentor. Explain what you hope to gain in a mentor-mentee partnership and what you may have to offer as well. Some people may feel honored, while others may be surprised, but they will almost always be willing to help a future nutrition professional in his or her career path.

References

1. Commission on Dietetic Registration. Introducing essential practice competencies. https://www.cdrnet.org/competencies. Accessed January 17, 2016.

2. Commission on Dietetic Registration. *Essential Practice Competencies for the Commission on Dietetic Registration's Credentialed Nutrition and Dietetics Practitioners.* https://admin.cdrnet.org/vault/2459/web/files/FINAL-CDR_Competency.pdf. Accessed January 17, 2016.

3. Commission on Dietetic Registration. Essential practice competencies information. https://www.cdrnet.org/essential-practice-competencies-information. Accessed January 17, 2016.

4. Commission on Dietetic Registration. Benefits of the professional development portfolio. https://www.cdrnet.org/pdp/benefits-of-the-professional-development-portfolio. Accessed January 17, 2016.

5. Commission on Dietetic Registration. Professional development portfolio. https://www.cdrnet.org/pdp/professional-development-portfolio-guide?preview=true. Accessed January 17, 2016.

6. Commission on Dietetic Registration. Frequently asked questions (FAQs) about the professional development portfolio (PDP). https://admin.cdrnet.org/vault/2459/web/files/Competencies%20FAQ.pdf. Accessed January 17, 2016.

7. Commission on Dietetic Registration. CPE offerings and resources. https://www.cdrnet.org/products/continuing-professional-development-education. Accessed January 17, 2016.

8. Academy of Nutrition and Dietetics. Professional development. http://www.eatrightpro.org/resources/career/professional-development. Accessed January 17, 2016.

9. US Department of Agriculture, National Agriculture Library. Professional and career resources. http://fnic.nal.usda.gov/professional-and-career-resources. Accessed January 17, 2016.

10. Academy of Nutrition and Dietetics. Academy groups. http://www.eatrightpro.org/resources/membership/academy-groups. Accessed January, 2016.

CHAPTER 7

Landing Your First Job . . . and Beyond

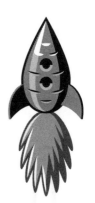

THOUGHT QUESTIONS

- Research entry-level job openings using the resources listed in this chapter or by searching online job databases. Identify three to five positions that appeal to you, along with the job description and academic requirements.

- Using resources from the Commission on Dietetic Registration (CDR), describe a few ways to obtain continuing professional education (CPE) units. Be specific, providing examples of opportunities that are currently available.

- Although it might seem far away now, depending on where you are in your education or career, envision what you want to achieve in the next 5 to 10 years and write down three possible goals. These may include thoughts on starting your own business or obtaining a specialty certification or advanced degree.

GOOD NEWS! THE SAME SKILLS YOU USED TO LAND YOUR dietetic internship, such as obtaining strong recommendations, preparing for an interview, and putting together a winning application, will also help you find your first job as a registered dietitian nutritionist (RDN). Now, all you need is to do is update your resume, develop a cover letter, and polish your professional portfolio or marketing materials. Because there are many other general resources for job applicants (career centers, books, or online resources), this chapter will focus on information specific to the job hunt within the dietetics field.

Where Registered Dietitian Nutritionists Work

As you may recall from Chapter 1, about half of practicing registered dietitians nutritionists (RDNs) work in clinical settings, but there is a wide and diverse range of opportunities within the field of nutrition and dietetics. Macro trends, such as an increasingly aging population, growth in obesity and overweight (in both adults and children), high rates of chronic disease, and growing interest in food, fitness, and mobile health technology, have led to a greater need for RDNs in a variety of settings.

Before You Begin Your Job Search

Part of the exploration phase is to get an idea of the actual jobs that are out there. Browse online job postings and sign up for e-mail listserv job postings from your state affiliate, dietetic practice groups (DPGs), or student groups. If you know the company you want to work for, go directly to its career source or human resources department. Employers—including private companies or industries, universities, departments of health, and other government agencies—typically list job openings on their career websites. Read fully the job descriptions, education and experience requirements, and salary ranges. To learn about a wide variety of possible career paths within the field of nutrition and dietetics, check out a resource published by the Academy of Nutrition and Dietetics, *Job Descriptions: Models for the Dietetics Profession* (available from the eatrightSTORE, www.

eatrightstore.org). This offers sample job descriptions based on actual jobs and descriptions shared by practicing RDNs.

This initial exploration step will give you an idea of the job opportunities for you based on your experience. If you see a listing for your dream job, notice the road map of skills and experience you should work toward. But in the meantime, look for entry-level work that will help build the skills you need for the next step in your career.

JOB BANK WEBSITES

- CareerBuilder (www.careerbuilder.com)
- Idealist.org (www.idealist.org)
- iHireNutrition (www.ihirenutrition.com)
- Indeed (www.indeed.com)
- LinkedIn (www.linkedin.com)
- Monster (www.monster.com)
- Nutrition Jobs (www.nutritionjobs.com)

Tools for the Job Hunt

In a competitive job market, applicants must use all their assets to secure employment. Networking is one of the most important resources you can tap into to progress in your career. Your tangible tools for the job hunt are your resume, cover letter, professional portfolio, and marketing materials. You should also secure permission from three to four references to provide their contact information to prospective employers.

Networking

As we have used one or two clichés in this text already, it won't hurt to use another. **These days, and in this profession, it's all about who you know.** A large part of finding a job is having a network of contacts, which at this stage may include professors, internship preceptors, and previous employers or managers. Informational interviews are a great place to start building your network if you want to learn about a person or organization, especially if the person is doing the kind of job you find interesting. Ask about his or her career path, what a typical day is like in the job, and what skills or personality traits are necessary for the job. Learn what it would be like and what it would take to work within that setting, environment, or specialty field. This not only exposes you to potential employment settings but also gives employers a chance to meet you and learn about your skills and interests. It could even open up doors for future opportunities.

Meeting and then staying connected not only informs you of opportunities and updates in the field but also helps expand your viewpoint and knowledge of nutrition, and it may come in handy later when you need advice or help. Other ways to network are by volunteering for projects and dietetics-related events or attending lectures and conferences. If you are shy or nervous, practice your introduction for when you meet new people. Prepare about 10 to 30 seconds of information about yourself. It's not a monologue or an invitation to monopolize the conversation; it is really a moment to share key information about yourself, provide context and meaning behind who you are, and help people remember you later!

As you meet people, your aim should be to learn something about the person you're meeting and think about ways that you might connect in the future. For newcomers, networking is not about climbing some invisible ladder just to meet people and gain favors. Start by "putting in your time" and helping out others first. This could be serving on a committee, making an introduction, or offering advice to a student. That way, when you need something, others will be more likely to return the favor. Mentors are also a great source for networking opportunities (read more about setting up a mentor relationship in Chapter 6).

The Resume

Professionals should always have an updated resume ready. For students and recent graduates, a university career center usually

A Closer Look

Resume Tips from the Front Lines

At a staffing agency dedicated to registered dietitians, our eyes as recruiters scan a lot of resumes for similar positions. After only a short time as a recruiter, I've already picked up some insider information about how to make your resume stand out, and I want to share it.

The Words: Take a few minutes to dig into a posting's job description, and tailor your resume to it. Highlight the skills from your most recent positions that match up with the prospective position. Remove skills or sections of your resume that aren't relevant to the job. This will allow the necessary skills to shine.

Look for impact words in the job description and use those words (or similar ones) in your own resume if you have that experience. Words like "built," "directed," "assessed," and "solved" are all great action words. And be specific about how you used those skills. What did you build? How many did you direct? Include job description details from only your most recent and applicable positions. Leave out details from positions that ended more than 10 years ago. If you haven't practiced a skill in 10 years, chances are it shouldn't be included on your resume.

The Look: Consistency and chronology are key. Start your resume with your most recent/present position at the top. List the company, job title and dates you worked in the same order and format for each position. It doesn't matter if you use 8/1/2014 or August 1, 2014, just be consistent.

Font choice should be considered early. You want your resume to be memorable, but not for something negative. Stick with traditional fonts but use bold, italic and even shades of grey in the same font family to break up sections. It's an industry standard to keep your resume to one page, and font can help you reach this goal. Size 10-point font in Garamond takes up much less space than 10-point Arial. If you must use two pages, it's not a deal breaker, but don't go beyond two.

The Format: Your resume should come to the recruiters in an easy-open format. If you don't apply through our website and instead email your resume as an attachment, Word documents and PDFs are best. They automatically upload into our data system, which puts your information at our fingertips in seconds.

CONTINUED ›

A CLOSER LOOK (CONTINUED)

When you email a resume, consider the document name, email address, email subject, and email body. These will be seen before we even open the resume. Make sure to entice a recruiter, not confuse them. Remember, your resume represents your skills and credibility. Look at everything you're sending as a whole package and make sure to represent yourself well.

Excerpt from a blog article published July 2015 by Heidi Williams, recruiter at Dietitians on Demand, an RD/RDN staffing company that provides contract and permanent placement services in clinical and community settings. Used with permission.

provides resume review services and can help you craft a strong resume. Your internship director, professor, or mentor are other resources, as are many other general career or job applications guides.

The Cover Letter

Your cover letter is a chance to show your potential employer that you are an effective and professional communicator. Our tips on how to write a great cover letter are similar to our tips for a winning resume: Keep it short, informative, and professional, and tailor it to each job opportunity. Explain why you are applying for this specific job, and provide a few reasons why you would be the best fit, above other candidates. An example cover letter, as well as sample resumes, can be found on the Academy of Nutrition and Dietetics Career resources page (http://www.eatrightpro.org/resources/career).[1]

Marketing Materials

We recommend business cards and stationery that present you and your services in a professional manner. But no tap-dancing broccoli or apples with shades unless it fits your brand! Create a positive and professional image in all that you do. For great design-it-yourself services, we recommend (and use) Vistaprint (www.vistaprint.com) or Overnight Prints (www.overnightprints.com).

Work Samples

You may consider putting together a packet of your past work that is most relevant to the position at hand. This demonstrates not only your experience and expertise in the tasks that might be asked of you but also your preparation and organizational abilities. For example, if you're applying for a position in community health education, you might provide copies of past educational handouts or lesson plans that you've created. For a media spokesperson position, you might provide published writing samples or video segments, whereas for a health advocacy role, you might provide copies of a congressional testimony or a press release from a grassroots event you helped organize. The career or professional portfolio is one way to present this information, among your other qualifications and certifications, resume, and so forth.

BUILDING A PROFESSIONAL PORTFOLIO

For additional guidance on putting together a resume, check out our other book, *Creating Your Career Portfolio: At-a-Glance Guide for Dietitians* (Prentice Hall, 2004), which focuses on steps in building career portfolios. The career portfolio is a personalized compilation of all your qualifications, accomplishments, work samples, skills, and abilities. The career portfolio is an invaluable tool for the job application process, so we take you through the steps in planning, building, and using it effectively. Today, the e-portfolio, which is essentially an online or digital version of your professional portfolio, has become popular.

The Interview

When you've been invited for an interview, you're one step closer to landing a job, but the work is not over. It shows that your resume and cover letter sufficiently impressed a prospective employer, and now they're interested in learning more about you to see if you may be a good fit for their organization. There are many resources available to help you prepare for an interview, so we won't cover this in depth here. Just be prepared to answer different types of questions, especially the standard ones, such as "Tell me about yourself" or "What interests you about this job?" Many interviewers may also include questions that ask you to talk about an experience or situation where you had to utilize certain skills, such as critical thinking, problem solving, or conflict management. It's a good idea to review many types of potential interview questions and jot down possible answers so that you're prepared for the interview. Last piece of advice: Be sure that you have questions to ask the interviewer. This shows that you did your homework and researched the job and the employer in advance. The answers you receive and your overall experience help you decide if the potential employer is right for you as well!

ACCOUNTING FOR GAPS IN TIME

If your resume contains gaps in time, be prepared to explain why those gaps occurred. Employers may ask. Perhaps you took time off to raise a family, to further your education, or because you had a personal problem. Try to keep it positive, and be honest, but avoid oversharing any personal or unnecessary information.

The Salary Negotiation

Many people consider the salary negotiation to be their least favorite part of the job interview process. Remember that you have valuable, specialized skills and should be fairly compensated. In fact, not demanding fair compensation hurts the profession as a whole. But it's important to have a realistic perspective. Remember the field and organization you are negotiating with, the type of work you will be doing, where you will fit in the hierarchy, and the level of responsibility you will hold. Two smart, capable RDNs may find themselves with very different compensation depending on these factors. The goal in salary negotiation is getting a competitive compensation package relative to the type of job you're doing and the environment you're doing it in.

Speaking with your peers and mentors can provide a perspective on the going rate. Other resources include the Bureau of Labor Statistics, which offers information on salary percentiles for dietitians and nutritionists online and in its *Occupational Outlook Handbook*, and the Academy of Nutrition and Dietetics "Compensation and Benefits Survey of the Dietetics Profession," which is updated every two years and available free to members or for online purchase through the eatrightSTORE (www.eatrightSTORE.org).

Remember: Be bold! If you don't ask, you won't get. In your negotiations, wait to talk money until the company or employer mentions it first, which will typically be after an employment offer is extended. Let them make the first proposal so you have an idea of their position and can work from there to advocate for yourself.

Looking Ahead: Giving Back to the Profession

After you have landed yourself a paying job and have taken some time to get acclimated to your baseline time commitments, the next step is looking for ways to go above and beyond. If you plan to make a difference in your career, enjoy your job, become successful, earn a respectable living, and connect with others, we strongly encourage volunteering. Even the most talented or knowledgeable RDNs will benefit from and enjoy more success by taking part in the profession through volunteer opportunities.

Volunteering

To us, "getting involved" means reaching out beyond your daily job requirements or schoolwork and contributing your time to the food and nutrition community. You may become active at your district level (local association), affiliate (state association), national association (Academy of Nutrition and Dietetics), or within a DPG or member interest group (MIG). Becoming a preceptor for future students or getting involved with public policy and advocacy are other ways to give back. Here are other steps to get involved:

- In Academy of Nutrition and Dietetics groups (state affiliates, DPGs, or MIGs), there may be opportunities to serve on committees, such as the membership, public relations, event planning, or outreach committees. These roles can require varying commitment levels, whether you have 2 or 10 hours a week to offer, and can be a great way to start and often lead to more opportunities.
- Volunteering to help with fundraising is another important function, as dietetic associations often are looking to raise funds for scholarships, political action committees, and conference expenses, among other things.
- If you enjoy your work on any given committee, consider applying for a leadership position, such as committee leader or chair or executive committee position (president, vice president, secretary, treasurer, and so on). We recommend waiting for this step until you've gained a more sufficient experience—this way, you'll know what you're committing to and will have gathered contacts to help you get nominated and elected.

Our best advice is this: Never hesitate to reach out! When looking for opportunities, try e-mailing the president, membership chair, or other members in leadership positions. Organizations are always looking for extra help, and they will be grateful for and glad to see your interest. Additionally, past professors, employers, or other mentors are also resources to offer advice, ideas, and new connections. So throw your hat in the ring with an e-mail or phone call. You never know how many doors will open down the road, not to mention what you will learn.

Calling All Preceptors!

Volunteering to be a preceptor is one of the most rewarding ways to make a difference in the future of the profession. In this role, you will act as a mentor, helping train and educate dietetics students. If more practitioners are willing to take on this role, it can help expand the availability of dietetic internships. For individuals who are interested, the Commission on Dietetic Registration (CDR) has even created an online preceptor training course, which qualifies for eight CPE units.[2] Furthermore, to facilitate connections between students and available preceptors, the Accreditation Council for Education in Nutrition and Dietetics (ACEND) offers a database, called "Find-a-Preceptor," where practitioners can register to become preceptors.[3] This database allows program directors and students to search for a preceptor by geographical or specialty area.

FINDING WORK-LIFE BALANCE

Striking a healthy balance in your professional and personal lives is an important step in growing professionally. It requires planning and effective time management. Map out your calendar or schedule and set aside time for the things you need to get done. Then look to see where you might have extra time for volunteering or other activities.

Another step is learning how far you can stretch yourself without impairing work performance and personal relationships. Failing to complete tasks as best you can will also reflect poorly on you, so accept responsibility for volunteer activities only if you know it's possible. Otherwise, pass on the opportunity, recommend names of a couple of other people who may be a good fit, and wait for the next time you can help. Ultimately, knowing when to say "no" is as important as knowing when to say "yes."

Your Voice in Public Policy

Public policy and advocacy is another opportunity for students and RDNs to advance the profession and have their voices heard. Through both the Academy of Nutrition and Dietetics efforts and individual efforts, the field of nutrition and dietetics has made significant advances in legislative activities over the past decade. As of 2015, the Academy of Nutrition and Dietetics has identified three priority areas for policy: (1) disease prevention and treatment, (2) life cycle nutrition, and (3) quality health care. More information about each of these areas can be found on the Academy of Nutrition and Dietetics "Advocacy" page on its website.[4]

For those looking to get involved in professional advocacy, the Academy of Nutrition and Dietetics provides many resources, including information on bills, laws, and regulations; public policy workshops and tips for success in advocacy; and regular updates on new legislation. The Academy of Nutrition and Dietetics also has its own political action committee (PAC; the Academy of Nutrition and Dietetics is called ANDPAC), which collects financial contributions from members and then allocates the pooled resources to support political candidates who are pronutrition, profood, and prohealth, and may support issues such as insurance coverage for nutrition services, food assistance programs, and hunger issues. ANDPAC is ranked among the top health professional political action committees and supports an Academy-led policy and advocacy team in Washington, DC.

Working with the Media and Getting Published

RDNs have a lot to offer the media as expert sources for scientifically sound nutrition and health information. Many major magazines and online publications have RDNs as writers or on their editorial boards. Journalists and news anchors rely on the expertise of RDNs frequently for interpretation of the latest research findings, tips on diet and lifestyle, and food or recipe suggestions (to name a few topics). In this way, the media offer RDNs an opportunity to disseminate advice and educate the public on a larger scale. Media engagement promotes the profession too.

So how can you get involved? Individuals who excel in media work can apply to be one of the Academy of Nutrition and Dietetics spokespeople—registered dietitians representing the largest media markets and specialty nutrition areas—and function as the media's best resource for expert commentary, story ideas, and background on a full range of food and nutrition topics.[5] The selection process is rigorous and requires experience, so it's a good goal to aim for if you're interested in working with the media. Even if you are not an Academy media spokesperson, you can still send your information to local editors and producers, along with a headshot (photo), resume,

A Closer Look

Communicating the Science of Nutrition and the Art of Good Food

People are hungrier than ever for realistic options that empower them to make healthier choices while bringing back the enjoyment of food. RDNs are qualified to help people separate science fiction from science fact and come away with meaningful steps toward better nutrition and health. By embracing and creating nutrition communication opportunities in the media, dietitians can branch out to a larger audience for more reach, visibility, and impact.

Unfortunately, the loudest voices in the media are not always the most credible. How often do we hear oversimplified, sensationalized, fear-mongering misinformation from celebrities and other "experts"? It is crucial that more dietitian voices are heard in the media so that credible, meaningful nutrition information and advice dominates the conversation. If we aren't part of the conversation, we cannot be part of the solution!

As RDNs, we have our work cut out for us, compared to celebrity "experts" and fear-mongers who say whatever they want. We must be clear, concise and compelling while still being evidence-based. We need to provide real solutions for real people so they can enjoy their food with health in mind.

Here are my top tips for effective, engaging and empowering communication:

1. Strive to create food and nutrition messages that include these three components:
   - sound science (evidence-based)
   - smart nutrition (realistic, meaningful, creative solutions; not boring or vague)
   - good food (savor and celebrate food; simple cooking or trying a new recipe; no fear factors)

2. Make sure your messages possess what I call the **"OOOh!"** factor:
   - your information is **O**rganized so it is more memorable and meaningful
   - your messages are **O**riginal because they are in your own words and your personality shines
   - you provide tangible takeaways that make your audience say **"Oh**, I can do that!"

CONTINUED ›

A CLOSER LOOK (CONTINUED) ···

The media landscape continues to evolve, providing RDNs with new op-portunities to highlight their expertise, while promoting RDNs as *the* nutrition experts. Traditional media (TV, radio and print) opportunities are shrinking while digital ones are expanding. Videos, podcasts, and self-publishing are just a few strategic alternatives that allow RDNs to embrace their inner "celebrity" and gain valuable exposure.

Ultimately, RDNs must have a powerful voice in *all* types of nutrition communication—media, social media, public speaking, writing, blog-ging, podcasting, and more. Dietitians with excellent communication skills have more career opportunities, more job satisfaction, and higher income than dietitians with technical skills alone. Top communicators have more influence in their organization, are more effective with pa-tients or clients, negotiate better raises or benefits, and have more visi-bility in their communities.

By Melissa Joy Dobbins, MS, RDN, CDE, The Guilt-Free RD—"Because food shouldn't make you feel bad!" and CEO of Sound Bites, Inc. Sound Science. Smart Nutrition. Good Food (www.soundbitesRD.com).

and biographical sketch of your expertise and accomplishments, and let them know you're available for interviews. This is a great way to get media experience.

If you wish to write for certain publications, check their web-sites for tips and instructions for potential writers. Look for infor-mation on contacting editors, writing styles and formatting, and the submittal and review process and timing. If you haven't published anything substantial, start with local or college newspapers, hospital or DPG newsletters, regional magazines, and online blogs or forums. Although the pay may be minimal or nonexistent, this work builds published samples of your writing (clips) to show future editors.

As you gain experience, check out *Writer's Market* (Writer's Di-gest Books), which is published annually and available online, and provides information on editors, the magazines they work for, and

MEDIA TIPS

Stay informed about local and national news and nutrition research. Read peer-reviewed journals and subscribe to the Academy's e-mail updates, such as the *Daily News* or *Eat Right Weekly*. It's important that you can translate nutrition research into explanations, advice, or recommendations that the average person will understand.

Be prepared when the media call. Journalists are looking for succinct answers to their questions. Know your subject, stay focused on a few key messages, give concise answers, and tailor your speaking to fit the audience. Concentrate on "teaching points" rather than a lengthy discussion.

Practice dealing with the unexpected. An interviewer may stray from the subject at hand or ask additional and unrelated questions. Prepare a few statements that help get back on topic.

Start a database of your media contacts. This includes name, company, address, telephone number, and e-mail. After a media interview, whether by phone, radio, or television, make notes of what was said and done. Send a thank-you e-mail. Keep copies of all interviews and media clips and add these to your resume and professional portfolio.

the types of articles they are looking for. When you are ready to make contact, develop a pitch letter that opens with an interesting fact or attention-grabbing statement to demonstrate just how fascinating you are! The next paragraph should explain precisely and in detail what you propose for the article. To close, describe yourself, your credentials, and your experience. Provide complete contact information and timing for when you will follow up. It may take up to several months to hear back.

A Final Word: Ethics in Dietetics

We thought we would end this chapter with a note about ethics—a principle that is inherent within the dietetics and nutrition profession. The Academy of Nutrition and Dietetics and CDR have implemented an official Code of Ethics, which provides guidance to dietetics practitioners in their professional practice and conduct.[6] The fundamental principles of the Code of Ethics are that dietetics practitioners will (1) "conduct themselves with honesty, integrity and fairness" and (2) "support and promote high standards of professional practice by reporting perceived violations of the Code of Ethics."[6] The Code of Ethics was created not only to guide the practice of nutrition and dietetics but also for the interest of the public we serve. It applies to all dietetics practitioners, including all Academy of Nutrition and Dietetics members and all CDR-credentialed dietetics practitioners.

References

1. Academy of Nutrition and Dietetics. Resume templates. http://www.eatrightpro.org/resource/career/career-development /career-toolbox/resume-templates. Accessed January 17, 2016.

2. Commission on Dietetic Registration. CDR's online campus. http://www.cdrcampus.com. Accessed January 17, 2016.

3. Accreditation Council for Education in Nutrition and Dietetics. Preceptors or mentors. http://www.eatrightacend.org/ACEND /content.aspx?id=6442464994. Accessed January 17, 2016.

4. Academy of Nutrition and Dietetics. Advocacy. http://www .eatrightpro.org/resources/advocacy. Accessed January 17, 2016.

5. Academy of Nutrition and Dietetics. Spokespeople. http://www .eatrightpro.org/resources/media/meet-our-spokespeople /spokespeople. Accessed January 17, 2016.

6. Academy of Nutrition and Dietetics. Code of Ethics. http://www .eatrightpro.org/resources/career/code-of-ethics. Accessed January 17, 2016.

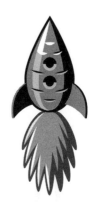

CHAPTER 8

Movers and Shakers

THROUGHOUT THIS BOOK, WE HAVE FOCUSED ON PRO-
viding you with the essential information you need to become
a dietitian and succeed in your chosen career. Now it's time
to take an inside look at the profession of nutrition and dietetics. We
are pleased to introduce you to just a few of the movers and shakers
of our profession in a variety of specialty areas. These folks know
how to work well with others, build influential alliances, and function
as savvy businesspeople. They are trailblazers, taking their careers
to the next level by doing all of the things we've described in this
book—and more. In fact, many will have moved on to new adven-
tures and accomplishments by the time this is published. And, by the
way, many of these people inspired us in our careers!

Read on to learn the unique career pathways, accomplishments, and words of wisdom from several of the many ambitious and successful registered dietitian nutritionists (RDNs) and registered dietitians (RDs).*

Communication: Liz Marr, MS, RDN, FAND

Claim to Fame

Liz Marr, the principal and founder of Liz Marr and Associates, LLC, in Longmont, CO, is a food and nutrition communication expert with nearly 30 years of experience in the field of food, nutrition, and culinary arts. Liz specializes in scientific and consumer writing, recipe development, and nutrition information analysis. A veteran media resource and spokesperson, she has participated in nearly 1,000 media interviews. Her current passions are combining science and art to produce highly valued deliverables for clients, serving as a role model for other food and nutrition professionals, and balancing professional and personal life. In 2014, she became a fellow of the Academy of Nutrition and Dietetics (the Academy). She has also been recognized by the Colorado Dietetic Association as Outstanding Dietitian of the Year, and Recognized Young Dietitian of the Year prior to that.

Education and Training

Liz received a master of science in food and nutrition science from Colorado State University and a bachelor of science from University of Missouri, Columbia, in family and consumer sciences, specializing in fashion merchandising. Her entrepreneurial ventures started in 2000 when she was cofounder and principal of Marr Barr Communications, LLC, a women- and RD-owned public relations (PR) firm specializing in food, nutrition, environment, and agriculture,

---

* The RDN and RD credentials are interchangeable, legally protected titles. Only dietetics professionals who have completed the requirements outlined in previous chapters can call themselves an RDN or RD—credentials that represent competence to provide services to patients and clients. The RDN credential was offered as an option, beginning in 2013, to RDs who want to emphasize the nutrition aspect of their credential to the public and to other health practitioners.

including natural and organic products. Earlier on in her career, Liz was manager of consumer communication for Horizon Organic Dairy in Boulder, CO, and vice president of programs for the Western Dairy Council and Western Dairy Farmers Promotion Association.

Giving Back to the Profession

Liz explains, "I have had the good fortune to have the support of numerous mentors in the field. It was a former boss, the Colorado Dietetic Association president at the time, who referred me to the local Dairy Council, where I started my first full-time position after graduate school. I stayed with the Dairy Council for 12 years before moving on to Horizon Organic Dairy and then colaunching a successful PR firm with another RD.

"The choice to be self-employed has allowed me the independence and flexibility to balance my personal and professional endeavors and has been immensely rewarding."

With her successes, Liz also believes, "What goes around comes around: Volunteer and nurture those around you—you will gain far more than you give." Through the years, she has actively supported the dietetics profession, serving as an Academy spokesperson and in the following positions:

- Chair, Food and Culinary Professionals dietetic practice group (DPG)
- Chair, Nutrition Education for the Public DPG
- Board of Trustees member, Society for Nutrition Education Foundation
- Chair, Nutrition and Food Science Section of the International Association of Culinary Professionals
- President, Colorado Dietetic Association

Liz Marr's Words of Wisdom

Make friends, ask questions, strive for high-quality performance, set your boundaries, and charge what you are worth.

Internet Communication: Kathleen M. Zelman, MPH, RD

Claim to Fame

Kathleen Zelman is a nutrition and communication consultant. Currently, she works in private practice in Atlanta, GA, specializing in food, health, and nutrition communication for consumer and health professional audiences. She is director of nutrition for one of the world's largest online health and wellness websites and is the nutrition expert for United Healthcare's Source 4 Women, where she serves as an editor, recipe developer, and nutrition communicator to educate consumers on news and trends in food and nutrition. Kathleen works through different types of media: articles, blogs, webinars, and videos. In the past, she has partnered with chefs Emeril Lagasse and Paul Prudhomme and has consulted with media outlets including CNN, *Good Morning America*, *NBC Nightly News*, *CBS Evening News*, *World News*, the *Wall Street Journal*, and the *New York Times*.

Education and Training

With over 30 years of experience, Kathleen's training includes a master's degree in public health from Tulane University and a bachelor of science from Montclair State University in New Jersey. Previously, she has worked as a clinical dietitian and in private practice, as an instructor at Georgia State University and an assistant professor of nutrition at St. Mary's Dominican College, and as the dietetic internship director at Ochsner Medical Institutions.

Giving Back to the Profession

Kathleen observes, "Throughout my career, I have firmly believed in giving back to my profession. On a local, state, and national level, I have held numerous offices and positions. It is with great pleasure that I volunteer to serve the profession, and I must admit, the networking and friendships that have grown from my volunteer work are the greatest rewards."

In addition to serving 12 years as an Academy media spokesper-son, Kathleen's other contributions have included the following:

- State media representative, Louisiana Dietetic Association
- Director-at-large, Academy of Nutrition and Dietetics Board of Directors
- Georgia delegate, Academy of Nutrition and Dietetics House of Delegates
- Past trustee, Georgia Dietetic Foundation

Kathleen Zelman's Words of Wisdom

Follow your dreams and challenge yourself to always learn and grow to expand your skills in our science-driven profession.

If you love what you do, you will be rewarded with a fabulous career and the great satisfaction that comes from helping others.

Say yes when you want to say no. Taking risks is the greatest way to reach your potential.

Clinical Informatics: Pam Charney, PhD, RD

Claim to Fame

Pam Charney is the program chair of the health care informatics baccalaureate degree at Bellevue College in Washington, where she hopes to develop informatics competencies for training RDNs in the future. She is responsible for program curriculum and learning outcomes, budget, program integrity, and course development and evaluation. As an expert consultant on electronic health records, Pam has a unique focus on adolescent access to personal health records. Notably, Pam was the first dietitian selected to receive a National Library of Medicine fellowship for the Biomedical Informatics Short Course and was invited to the 2006 Nursing Technology Informatics Guiding Education Reform (TIGER) meeting. Other awards include:

- Academy of Nutrition and Dietetics Medallion Award
- Academy of Nutrition and Dietetics Award for Excellence in

Clinical Nutrition

- Dietitians in Nutrition Support DPG Distinguished Dietitian Award
- American Society for Parenteral and Enteral Nutrition (A.S.P.E.N.) Outstanding Nutrition Support Dietitian Award

Pam also participates in leadership activities for the American Medical Informatics Association (AMIA). She has been a member of AMIA's Education Committee and is now a member of the Member ship/Outreach and Working Group Steering Committees.

Education and Training

Pam has extensive training in clinical nutrition care and informatics. She completed her undergraduate studies at the University of West Florida and dietetic internship at Walter Reed Army Medical Center. She earned her PhD at the University of Medicine and Dentistry of New Jersey, where she has been highlighted as an outstanding alumna. Pam also has a master's degree in clinical informatics and patient-centered technology from the University of Washington. Previously, Pam worked as a nutrition support dietitian, pediatric dietitian, and clinical nutrition manager at Madigan Army Medical Center and has gained more than 20 years of experience as a practitioner and manager in a variety of hospital settings.

Giving Back to the Profession

Pam observes, "I received a thank-you note from one of our program graduates, which said 'thanks for standing up for me and our profession.' This spoke volumes; I make it a point to teach students that if you've chosen this career, then you have to take the responsibility to stand up for your choice. To do so you have to not only possess a certain level of assertiveness but you also have to know your stuff."

Pam's contributions to dietetics are extensive; she has served in the following positions:

- Director, Academy of Nutrition and Dietetics House of Delegates
- Member, Academy of Nutrition and Dietetics Board of Directors
- Charter member, Academy of Nutrition and Dietetics Standardized Language Committee
- Member, Academy of Nutrition and Dietetics Research Committee
- Past chair and website manager, Dietitians in Nutrition Support DPG
- Board of Directors member, A.S.P.E.N.

Pam Charney's Words of Wisdom

"No one can make you feel inferior without your consent."—Eleanor Roosevelt, America's First Lady

Life is too short to be serious all the time—find something to laugh at every day

Nutrition Support: Marion F. Winkler, PhD, RD, CNSC

Claim to Fame

Marion Winkler is the surgical nutrition specialist at Rhode Island Hospital and an associate professor of surgery in the Alpert Medical School of Brown University. In her clinical role, Marion provides nutrition care for acute and critical care patients, as well as diet/ nutrition education for complex patient issues and home parenteral and enteral nutrition patients. As an associate professor, she develops and provides didactic and clinical nutrition education for many, including dietetic interns, medical students, residents, and fellows. Marion has published extensively on nutrition assessment, parenteral nutrition, and quality assurance in nutrition support practice, with a particular emphasis on using qualitative methods to assess the quality of life of home parenteral nutrition patients. With such breadth of experience and commitment to the profession, Marion has received numerous awards and accolades, most notably the following:

- Academy of Nutrition and Dietetics Medallion Award
- Lenna Frances Cooper Lecture at the Academy of Nutrition and Dietetics Food and Nutrition Conference Expo (2009)
- Distinguished Award in Nutrition Support Dietetics

Education and Training

Prior to gaining over 30 years of experience in nutrition support practice, Marion earned her bachelor of science in nutrition from Case Western Reserve University in Cleveland, OH; her master of science in allied health from the University of Connecticut; and a PhD in health sciences from Rutgers (formerly the University of Medicine and Dentistry of New Jersey).

Giving Back to the Profession

Marion notes, "I am indebted to the terrific role models I had as an undergraduate and graduate student. Not only did I gain knowledge and practical experience, I was exposed and encouraged to participate in professional association activities. Having attended three universities that were homes to former Academy presidents, it is not surprising that I have followed in their leadership footsteps! Professional volunteerism has become a way of life for me." Marion's own contributions to the profession are demonstrated by the following accomplishments:

- Chair, Dietitians in Nutrition Support DPG
- Delegate from Rhode Island, Academy of Nutrition and Dietetics House of Delegates
- Council on Professional Issues delegate for clinical nutrition, Academy of Nutrition and Dietetics House of Delegates
- First dietitian to serve as president of A.S.P.E.N.
- President and Board of Directors member, A.S.P.E.N. Rhoads Research Foundation
- Board of Trustees member, Oley Foundation

Marion Winkler's Words of Wisdom

Find good role models, and mentor others.

Listen carefully to what your patients tell you.

Culinary Nutrition: Jackie Newgent, RDN

Claim to Fame

Jackie Newgent is a self-employed culinary nutritionist based in Brooklyn, New York. She works as a cookbook author, culinary instructor, professional recipe developer, freelance writer, and media spokesperson. In her daily life, she develops original, healthful recipes for national media outlets, pitches culinary and nutrition stories to news media on behalf of food clients, and maintains a regular presence in social media platforms. Jackie has authored *Big Green Cookbook* (2009), *1,000 Low-Calorie Recipes* (2012), and the award-winning books *The All-Natural Diabetes Cookbook* (2007) and *The With or Without Meat Cookbook* (2014). In 2015, the second edition of *The All-Natural Diabetes Cookbook* was released. Her expertise has been featured on national talk shows and news programs, including *Good Morning America* and *Dateline*, as well as in major print and online publications including *Everyday with Rachael Ray* magazine and Livestrong.com.

Education and Training

With the credentials of both an RD and a classically trained chef, Jackie has completed the education and training for both professions. She received her bachelor of science in allied health professions from The Ohio State University and her certificate in professional cooking from Kendall College. Her career experience has been diverse, including corporate wellness programming, obesity counseling, rehabilitation center consulting, and healthy after-school programming. Visit her website (www.jackienewgent.com) to learn more about her current and past projects and experience as the Natural Culinary Nutritionist.

Giving Back to the Profession

Regarding giving back to the profession, Jackie believes that "a self-marketing key is my involvement with professional membership groups and associations, such as the Food and Culinary Professionals DPG. I was on their board for several years and wholeheartedly enjoyed the experience. I feel so lucky to have a career that's happily intertwined with my life."

In addition to this DPG experience, Jackie is a former national media spokesperson for the Academy. She also volunteers as a preceptor for dietetic interns, helping to train future registered dietitians.

Jackie Newgent's Words of Wisdom

Strive to find a way to include whatever you are truly passionate about into your career.

Keep following your dreams—even when you hit a couple "nightmares" along your journey.

Disordered Eating: Jessica Setnick, MS, RD, CEDRD

Claim to Fame

Jessica Setnick is a Texas-based dietitian specializing in eating disorders. Best known for her straightforward approach to treating eating disorders, Jessica is the owner of two online resources, www.understandingnutrition.com and www.eatingdisorderjobs.com; the founder of the Eating Disorders Boot Camp; and the author of *The Eating Disorders Clinical Pocket Guide* (2013) and two editions of the *Academy of Nutrition and Dietetics Practice Guide to Eating Disorders* (2011, 2016). She is currently a senior fellow for Remuda Ranch in Wickenburg, AZ, where she consults and provides staff training to keep the treatment program up to date with developments in the field. Nationwide, she speaks publicly to educate the professional community and gain awareness for eating disorder treatment. Through her work,

Jessica hopes to empower professionals in the eating disorders field with confidence, competence, and community and to use new technology to improve dietetics education in the treatment of eating disorders.

Education and Training

Jessica received her bachelor of arts from the University of Pennsylvania and completed a master of science in exercise physiology and sports nutrition and a dietetic internship at Texas Woman's University. She also carries multiple additional credentials, including a health promotion certification by the Cooper Institute for Aerobics Research and certification as a certified eating disorder specialist (CEDRD).

Giving Back to the Profession

Jessica states, "Being a dietitian has been incredibly rewarding and at times very trying. I have found that many people have a limited or incorrect view of dietitians. There are so many possibilities of careers, projects, and options once you have the degrees and qualifications. Today, my nutrition education was only the basis for what I do now. Everything since then I have learned through continuing education, seeking advisers, and reading up on the topics I need." Jessica also gives back to the profession as a member and leader of various organizations, including:

- Past chair, Behavioral Health Nutrition DPG
- Cofounder, in 2012, International Federation of Eating Disorder Dietitians (IFEDD)
- Member, International Association of Eating Disorder Professionals (IAEDP), and Addiction Professionals Resource Alliance
- CEDRD supervisor; creator of the first CEDRD prep class

Jessica Setnick's Words of Wisdom

If you know what you want to accomplish, ask people for advice that can get you there, not for their opinions on whether you should

If you are committed to your idea, you don't need anyone else's approval to go for it or anyone else's doubts to rain on your parade.

Your first job may not be your dream job, but you never know what opportunities will arise just by being "out there." So step into that first job with your whole heart and learn all you can so that when the

Extended Care / Assisted Living: Becky Dorner, RDN, LD, FAND

Claim to Fame

Becky Dorner is founder/president of Nutrition Consulting Services, Inc, whose dedicated team of RDNs and nutrition and dietetics technicians, registered (NDTRs) have served health care facilities in Ohio since 1983, and Becky Dorner & Associates, Inc, which provides a library of resources and continuing education programs on healthy aging and nutrition care for older adults. In both roles, Becky is the visionary, strategist, mentor, and coach to more than 30 staff members and associates. She coordinates the operational and financial aspects of the business, as well as human resources and marketing. With expertise in nutrition, aging, and long-term health care, Becky's mission is to empower health care professionals to improve the health of aging adults and improve nutrition care for older adults. She has presented at hundreds of professional meetings and conferences in five countries and all 50 states and has published more than 270 manuals, continuing education programs, and practical articles, as well as an electronic newsletter for health care professionals in the field. The following are a few of Becky's awards and honors:

- Academy of Nutrition and Dietetics Award of Excellence in Business and Consultation
- Academy of Nutrition and Dietetics Recognized Young Dietitian of the Year
- Dietetics in Health Care Communities Distinguished Member Award

- Nutrition Entrepreneurs DPG Outstanding Nutrition Entrepreneur

Education and Training

Becky obtained her undergraduate degree from the University of Akron in nutrition and dietetics. Her previous work experiences involve an array of settings, including acute care, outpatient counseling and group classes, home health care, and foodservice director. Much of her postgraduate education has come from learning what she needed to run two successful nutrition and dietetics–related businesses and volunteering for professional organizations.

Giving Back to the Profession

Becky notes, "My volunteer work has helped hone my speaking, writing, and leadership skills. I have made friends across the country and abroad, and I know experts in all areas of practice. Because of volunteer work with other national organizations, my network has expanded outside nutrition and dietetics to nurses, physicians, ancillary professionals, and entrepreneurs. I have been blessed to work with incredible role models, mentors, volunteer leaders, employees, and friends. Some of the wisest have taught me what was most important in the journey: joy, love, laughter, family, friends, fun, and good health."

With such an apparent passion and drive for the profession, her volunteer experience is extensive. A few examples include:

- Speaker of House of Delegates, Academy of Nutrition and Dietetics
- Member, Academy of Nutrition and Dietetics Executive Board of Directors and Board of Directors
- Chair, the Academy of Nutrition and Dietetics Council on Future Practice and Dietetics in Health Care Communities DPG
- Officer, National Pressure Ulcer Advisory Panel
- Member of various Academy committees, including the Member Services Advisory Committee, Finance and Audit Committee, Legislative and Public Policy Committee, Nutrition Care

Process and Standardized Language Committee, Research Committee, and Unintended Weight Loss in Older Adults Evidence Analysis Library Work Group

Becky Dorner's Words of Wisdom

Take the time to become clear on what it is you want from your career. Create a vision board and write your goals with time lines. Keep your goals where you can see them, and review often.

Find a mentor or coach to help you stay focused on achieving your goals.

Volunteer for your professional organization. It will help you achieve your goals, expand your skills and network, and most importantly, support the future of the profession.

Maintain balance between career and family—at the end of the day, what really matters is your health and your relationships with others.

Latino Nutrition: Malena Perdomo, MS, RD, CDE

Claim to Fame

Malena Perdomo is an adjunct professor of nutrition at Metropolitan State University of Denver, CO, and has community, clinical, and research experience. She is a nutrition consultant who works with companies, nonprofit organizations, and research programs to provide nutrition consultation and education. Malena is also a writer, recipe developer, and media spokesperson on both radio and television, serving six years as a spokesperson for the Academy and specializing in Latino nutrition. She coauthored a cookbook in Spanish, *Los Secretos de Maya* (2014), and English, *Maya's Secrets* (2012), based on a television health show during which Malena featured healthy Latin cuisine and gave nutrition advice. Learn more on her website (www.malenanutricion.com/en/).

Education and Training

Malena's dietetics training began when she undertook a government nutrition internship in Panama, which enabled her to become the 126th nutritionist in her country in 1995. She is a graduate of Florida State University–Panama Canal Branch and the University of Tennessee–Chattanooga. She also earned a master's degree from Rosalind Franklin University of Medicine and Science. In addition to being a registered dietitian, Malena is also a certified diabetes educator (CDE). Her prior job experiences include work for Kaiser Permanente Colorado, the Special Supplemental Nutrition Program for Women, Infants and Children (WIC) programs in Nashville and Denver, and community and research programs.

Giving Back to the Profession

Malena explains, "The dietetics profession has given me the chance to work in various positions and utilize my creativity and technical and media skills. I can't decide to do one thing in nutrition yet, because I love everything that I am doing. Helping people is what really motivates and drives my passion to teach others. I have made myself known as the Latin foods expert, but I am always learning something new. My patients come from all backgrounds and different countries. I feel that I take more from them than they take from me."

Malena served as the Latino nutrition spokesperson for the Academy from 2005 until 2011 and past chair of Latinos and Hispanics in Dietetics & Nutrition (LAHIDAN) member interest group.

Malena Perdomo's Words of Wisdom

Don't forget about Español! Being bilingual is fun and allows you to connect with and help more people. There are apps that can help improve your Spanish.

Beyond the language, cultural competence in nutrition involves learning about foods and ingredients of other cultures and knowing how to prepare them, especially traditional dishes.

When teaching in the community, I use a lot of visuals—such as food models, real foods, and food labels—and interactive group discussion, conversations, and experiential activities (eating is one of them).

Media and Nutrition: Carolyn O'Neil, MS, RDN, LD

Claim to Fame

Carolyn O'Neil is a notable nutrition expert, award-winning food writer, television personality, and president of O'Neil Nutrition Communications based in Atlanta, GA. Carolyn believes "the more you know, the more you can eat!" She's the author of *Southern Living*'s *Slim Down South Cookbook* (2013) and coauthor of the award-winning book *The Dish on Eating Healthy and Being Fabulous!* (2009). Carolyn writes a weekly food and lifestyle column for the *Atlanta Journal-Constitution*, called "Healthy Eating"; contributes food and travel features to *The Atlantan* and to *Atlanta Homes & Lifestyle Magazine*; and publishes her own blog, *O'NeilOnEating.com*. She appears on NBC *Atlanta & Company* with live weekly segments on food, nutrition, and cuisine and as the Lady of the Refrigerator nutrition expert on the Food Network series *Good Eats*.

Education and Training

Carolyn's master's degree in nutrition and communication is from Boston University, and her undergraduate degree in foods and nutrition is from Florida State University. During her career reporting for CNN on food, nutrition, and cuisine, Carolyn earned three James Beard Foundation Awards, and she was the first dietitian to be inducted into the James Beard Who's Who in Food and Beverage. The American Heart Association, Academy of Nutrition and Dietetics, Institute of Food Technologists, American Society for Nutrition, and National Restaurant Association have also presented Carolyn with awards for food and nutrition communication.

Giving Back to the Profession

Carolyn says, "Each time I tell someone I am a registered dietitian, I enjoy seeing their reaction. Through the years, the responses and the facial expressions have changed. In the 1980s, when I first started practicing, people would ask, 'What's that? Is that like a nutritionist?' And I'd have to go through some long explanation. . . . Being a dietitian at a dinner party was like being a minister in a bar! Jump forward to now. It's amazing when I say I'm a registered dietitian and the majority respond, 'Oh, that's really great,' then launch into questions about personal diet needs. Dietitians have emerged with a new image as nutrition experts who are food savvy and ready to share valuable and trustworthy personalized diet advice."

Carolyn O'Neil's Words of Wisdom

"Make it simple. Make it memorable. Make it inviting to look at. Make it fun to read." —Leo Burnett, advertising icon

Focus on what people want to know before you begin telling them what you think they should know.

If you enjoy what you're doing, it's not work. It's play.

Nutrition Support: Mandy L. Corrigan, MPH, RD, LD, CNSC, FAND

Claim to Fame

Mandy Corrigan is a nutrition support dietitian and a member of the Coram Home Nutrition Support Team in St. Louis, MO. In her role, she manages the safe delivery of home parenteral nutrition and serves as a clinical mentor/preceptor to newly hired RDNs. She also conducts clinical research and lectures nationally on topics related to parenteral nutrition. Mandy has contributed to various professional publications, including peer-reviewed journal articles, book chapters, a textbook, and newsletter publications. Mandy has received numerous awards for excellence, leadership, and research, including:

- 2015 Coram/CVS Dietitian of the Year
- 2014 A.S.P.E.N. Abstracts of Distinction
- 2013 Oley Foundation Home Parenteral Nutrition Research Prize
- 2012 A.S.P.E.N. Distinguished Service Award

Education and Training

Mandy's undergraduate degree is from Bowling Green State University in Bowling Green, OH. Her dietetic internship was completed at MetroHealth Medical Center in Ohio, and her master of public health is from Cleveland State University/Northeast Ohio Medical University. Prior to her current position, Mandy worked on the nutrition support team at Cleveland Clinic and as an intensive care unit dietitian at MetroHealth Medical Center.

Giving Back to the Profession

Mandy observes, "Volunteering for professional organizations pays dividends. It has been rewarding both professionally and personally. Giving time to our profession gives me a stronger commitment to dietetics, incredible networking opportunities, leadership skills, and lifelong friendships with RDNs around the country I likely would not have met otherwise. Organizations often are looking for volunteers, so don't hesitate to reach out to leaders in the group—they need your talents!"

As a leader in the field of nutrition support, Mandy has served in numerous leadership roles for the Academy's Dietitians in Nutrition Support DPG, A.S.P.E.N., and state-level nutrition organizations:

- Dietitians in Nutrition Support DPG: chair-elect, *Support Line* editor, and member of Strategic Planning and Advance Practice Residency Committees
- Exam Writing Committee—Academy/CDR and the National Board of Nutrition Support Certification
- A.S.P.E.N.: Home and Alternate Site Care Section chair; Home

and Alternate Care Standards Taskforce member; Sustain Operations Advisory Committee member; Home Parenteral Clinical Guideline Committee member

- Reviewer, *Journal of Parenteral and Enteral Nutrition*
- Secretary, Missouri/Southern Illinois Society for Parenteral and Enteral Nutrition

Mandy Corrigan's Words of Advice

I credit my success to exceptional mentors, teamwork with co-investigators, and a strong personal drive to contribute to areas where little research exists.

Find a mentor to help guide you, learn from, and gain constructive feedback from. Your mentor may change as you progress through different stages of your career. Pay it forward, and mentor others.

Seize every opportunity to educate members of the medical team about the interventions we offer as RDNs. Foundational pillars are visibility, communication with physicians, and patient advocacy.

Media and Fitness: Felicia D. Stoler, DCN, MS, RDN, FACSM, FAND

Claim to Fame

A registered dietitian and exercise physiologist, Dr. Felicia Stoler is a sought-after nutrition and fitness expert. On a yearly basis, she makes hundreds of appearances at conferences, on TV, and in radio, newspapers, magazines, and blogs. She is a part-time lecturer at Rutgers University in the Exercise Science Department and has a private practice, Felicia Stoler & Associates, in Red Bank, NJ, with three RDNs. Across all of this work, Felicia's main function is translating nutrition science into consumer-friendly terminology—whether it's for students, patients, or media. She also spends time traveling to learn firsthand where our food actually comes from and to better understand various aspects of the food we eat. This has helped her answer questions on new or controversial topics of nutrition and health, culinary, agricultural, and manufacturing practices.

Education and Training

Felicia joined the health and wellness field after a career at ABC News in New York City, before which she worked as a paralegal. She holds a double master's degree in nutrition and exercise physiology from Teachers College at Columbia University as well as a doctorate in clinical nutrition from Rutgers School of Health Related Professions, where her research in worksite wellness demonstrated the ability for a weekly nutrition and physical activity intervention to improve health outcomes. Her previous experiences are diverse. She was an adjunct professor at Brookdale Community College, host of the second season of TLC's *Honey We're Killing the Kids!*, and nutrition coordinator for the ING New York City Marathon. Her media experience has included work with Ovaltine, *Dateline,* NBC's first *Weight Loss Challenge*, Nike, GNC, Unilever, Cargill, the Florida Department of Citrus, Nesquik, Eli Lilly, Milk Pep, the National Dairy Council, Sirius Satellite Radio, Walt Disney Imagineering, and more.

Giving Back to the Profession

Felicia states, "I often say to others, consider how you measure success—is it money, personal satisfaction, how your peers perceive you, or your impact on society? For me, they are all important. I have worked hard to get everything I have achieved, but it is definitely tough balancing a career and family. While I am confident in my knowledge base, we must stay current with the research in our field and in other health-related disciplines. I am very lucky that I love what I do! Every day is different, and, above all, I am passionate about my work—and it shows."

Felicia's commitment to volunteering is an example of her passion, including:

- Fellow, American College of Sports Medicine (ACSM), and President (as well as other offices) of the Greater New York chapter of ACSM

- Member of four national ACSM committees: Health & Science Policy, Public Information & Communication, Exercise Is Medicine (Communication), and Task Force for Healthy Air Travel
- Nutritionist, City Harvest's NYC Marathon team, and for the New Jersey Council on Physical Fitness and Sports
- Delegate, Academy of Nutrition and Dietetics
- President, New Jersey Dietetic Association

Felicia Stoler's Words of Wisdom

Create your own opportunities. Over 18 years ago when I pondered my career change, I could never have imagined that I would be doing what I am doing now. Be open to change, and listen to your heart. If you don't love what you are doing—find something else!

Nutrition and exercise are the least expensive, least invasive, and most effective ways to prevent diseases.

Give back to the community; a candle loses nothing by lighting other candles.

Publishing: Regina Ragone, MS, RDN

Claim to Fame

Regina Ragone is food director for *Family Circle* magazine at Meredith Publishing in New York. She brings more than 25 years of nutrition expertise to the magazine, prior to which she was vice president of nutrition at Hunter Public Relations. Her primary responsibilities are leading the overall strategy for the food pages of *Family Circle*, collaborating with colleagues in the food department to develop various food features, and writing and editing food pages. She is author of *Win the Fat War* (2001) cookbook and *Decadent Diabetic Desserts* (2003) and coauthor of *Meals That Heal* (2001). Currently, she resides on Long Island, where she enjoys her vegetable garden and experimenting in the kitchen.

Education and Training

Regina received her master's degree in nutrition from Queens College and her bachelor's in nutrition and foods from New York University. In addition to *Family Circle*, her other publishing positions have included an internship at *Restaurant Business* magazine, food editor for *Prevention* magazine, food editor at *Weight Watchers* magazine and the Weight Watchers Publishing Group, and test kitchen director for *Ladies' Home Journal*. She also worked as an assistant manager of the Global Consumer Food Center of the Campbell Soup Company and a public school foodservice dietitian, and she was vice president at Ogilvy Public Relations.

Giving Back to the Profession

Regina notes, "I have worked with several consumer publications as well as a nutritionist for two public relations companies. Every time I made a change it was difficult, and there was always a learning curve. I have had to tap into many of the nutrition contacts I've made through the years to help me. I am grateful for all of the support from my colleagues in every step of my journey and am excited to see where we're all headed."

Regina is a member of the Academy and Les Dames d'Escoffier International, which is an invitational organization of women leaders in food, beverage, and hospitality whose mission is education and philanthropy. For both organizations, Regina often volunteers and shares her expertise at conferences and other events.

Regina Ragone's Words of Wisdom

Have a vision of where you want to go and write it down; I look back at the things I wrote down, and I have achieved them!

No one expects you to know everything, and others have more respect for you when you ask for their expertise.

Sports Nutrition: Julie H. Burns, MS, RD, CCN

Claim to Fame

Julie Burns is owner of SportFuel, Inc, a sports nutrition consulting company, and founder of Eat Like the Pros, a customized organic meal delivery service, located in Chicago, IL. Past and current clients include the Chicago Blackhawks, Chicago White Sox, Chicago Bears, Chicago Bulls, Northwestern University's varsity teams, Next Level Performance, high-level executives, and professional and elite athletes. Julie is currently working to bring a novel assessment tool she utilizes with her individual clients to the mass market, paired with customized supplements. This effort fits within her greater passion to provide personalized nutrition recommendations to optimize health, performance, and longevity.

Education and Training

Julie earned her bachelor's degree in nutrition and dietetics from the University of Illinois at Urbana-Champaign (1983) and a master's in clinical nutrition from the Massachusetts General Hospital Institute of Health Professions (1987). She is a registered and licensed dietitian in Illinois and is a board-certified clinical nutritionist (CCN), with experience in integrative sports nutrition, functional nutrition, clinical research, public speaking, and public relations consulting.

Giving Back to the Profession

When reflecting on her career, Julie describes, "During college, a friend gave me *The Athlete's Kitchen* by Nancy Clark, a sports dietitian in Boston. I was so excited to read and learn of the link between nutrition and sports performance that I decided to apply to the combined internship/master's program at Massachusetts General Hospital where Nancy had completed her studies. When I finished my master's degree, I returned home to Chicago to work in clinical research with Dr. Michael Davidson, a cardiologist who was starting a research center. This is where I honed counseling, marketing, and budgeting skills that have been instrumental in my businesses today. Dr. Davidson knew I was passionate about sports nutrition and recommended me to the Chicago Blackhawks when they called for a referral."

Julie's contributions to the profession and volunteer experiences are diverse and include the following:

- Executive Committee member, Sports, Cardiovascular, and Wellness Nutrition (SCAN) DPG
- Member, SCAN and Dietitians in Integrative and Functional Medicine DPGs
- Member, the ACSM, and International & American Association of Clinical Nutritionists (IAACN), and the Weston A. Price Foundation
- Former member, Gatorade Sport Science Institute's Sports Nutrition Advisory Board

Julie Burns's Words of Wisdom

Join the Dietitians in Integrative and Functional Medicine DPG and seek additional training in functional nutrition, epigenetics, and using food to optimize health, performance, and longevity. Health starts in the gut, and together, the right foods, nutrients, and healthy bacteria form this foundation!

Supermarket Nutrition: Maggie Moon, MS, RD

Claim to Fame

Maggie Moon is the senior manager of Nutrition Communications for The Wonderful Company, a health-inspired food and beverage company in Los Angeles. Maggie provides thought leadership for health communication for The Wonderful Company's portfolio and oversees the development, management, and evaluation of branded and category nutrition communication programs. With a seat on the industry nonprofit board Nutrition Research and Education Foundation, Maggie also helps guide nutrition research and communication strategy for all tree nuts. She is author of *The Elimination Diet: A Personal Approach* to *Determining Your Food Allergies* (2014) and is currently working on her next book. She also writes for publications ranging from peer-reviewed journals to trade magazines and consumer publications, such as *Today's Dietitian, IDEA Fitness Journal, Nutrition Today*, Livestrong.com, CDiabetes.com, and other periodicals. She is often quoted in major outlets, such as *Health* magazine, WomensHealth-Mag.com, Yahoo! Health, *Men's Journal*, and CNN, to name a few.

Education and Training

Maggie holds a bachelor's degree in English from the University of California at Berkeley and a master's degree in nutrition and education from Columbia University Teachers College, where she also completed her dietetic internship and served as editor-in-chief of *Grapevine Student Newsletter* for the program in nutrition. Prior to working with The Wonderful Company, Maggie was the corporate nutritionist for the New York City–based online grocery retailer FreshDirect, where she promoted public health by helping customers find healthful foods in grocery stores. She has also been a nutrition educator at the City University of New York's Brooklyn College, Harlem RBI Afterschool Nutrition Workshops and a nutrition communication consultant to the USA Rice Federation, Tea Council of the USA, Unilever, FirstJuice, Cranberry Institute, and KIND.

Giving Back to the Profession

Maggie explains, "What I value most are the personal connections I have made with colleagues who are all working toward improving health and quality of life for people through good nutrition. I feel grateful to be part of a profession with a public good mission. It's also a profession that highly values mentorship. I do my part by making myself available to those who are interested in my non-traditional career path and very much enjoy referring RDNs for opportunities that are a good match for them. I also precept dietetic interns, and have created new staff roles for RDNs on my own team."

Beyond her mentorship and preceptor activities, Maggie also gives back to the dietetics profession as an involved member with the Academy and various DPGs. She has served on the board for the Greater New York Dietetic Association and on the executive committee and website task force for the SCAN DPG.

Maggie Moon's Words of Wisdom

Work on self-awareness of your leadership and communication styles. There are ways to demonstrate leadership at all levels. Training is available. Seek it. Registered dietitians are naturally positioned as teachers and coaches, so it's important to keep working on how to be effective.

Be confident in your knowledge and skills while being humble and open to others' expertise. Know your strengths while recognizing others' strengths so that you'll know how to build the right team for any project.

In practice, showing people that eating healthfully on a budget is a delicious and winning combination!

Nutrition Education and Outreach: Marisa Moore, MBA, RDN, LD

Claim to Fame

Marisa Moore is a registered dietitian nutritionist and owner of Marisa Moore Nutrition, a nutrition consulting service based in Atlanta, GA (http://marisamoore.com). Using a food-first, mostly plant-based approach, Marisa helps people eat better, one morsel at a time, by hosting group classes, writing and blogging, and developing healthful recipes. She also works as a consultant for small and large businesses, including food and nutrition start-ups, and a brand ambassador to promote great food and healthy habits. A former national spokesperson for the Academy, Marisa is a trusted food and nutrition expert and has appeared on and in major media outlets, including the *Today Show*, the *New York Times*, the *Wall Street Journal*, and the *Washington Post*, as well as making regular appearances on CNN. She is also contributing editor for *Food & Nutrition Magazine* and a *Huffington Post* blogger.

Education and Training

Marisa is a graduate of Georgia State University, where she completed her nutrition and dietetics training and also earned a master's degree in business administration. Marisa worked in a variety of roles before private practice. She was an outpatient dietitian and a corporate nutritionist for a restaurant chain, and she has managed the employee worksite nutrition program at the US Centers for Disease Control and Prevention, among other jobs. Always ready for new passport stamps, Marisa loves to explore new countries, but in her spare time, you might find her dancing salsa or on a jog with her dog.

Giving Back to the Profession

Marisa states, "Nutrition and dietetics marries my passions for food, science, and education. I became a registered dietitian nutritionist because of the plethora of options and opportunities in the field . . . there is never an excuse for boredom." Among the opportunities that keep her busy is service to the dietetics profession. This includes her nine years as an Academy spokesperson, which she believes was one of the best things for her career.

Starting in June 2015, Marisa began a three-year term on the Academy of Nutrition and Dietetics Nominating Committee. She has also served as president and nominating committee member for the Georgia Academy of Nutrition and Dietetics, as nominating committee member of the Nutrition Entrepreneurs DPG, and in various appointed and elected volunteer roles related to communication in dietetics. Marisa is a mentor and dietetic intern preceptor to future RDs, helping them realize opportunities to discover their voices in the increasingly crowded space of food and nutrition communication.

Marisa Moore's Words of Wisdom

Find your niche. The number of options available in the field of nutrition and dietetics is both a blessing and a curse. I've learned that the most successful RDs speak to a target audience and thrive, versus trying to be all things to all people.

Private Practice Nutrition: Cynthia Sass, MPH, MA, RD, CSSD

Claim to Fame

Cynthia Sass is a three-time *New York Times* best-selling author and nationally known nutrition expert and health educator. She has been quoted or made appearances in dozens of national publications, radio shows, and television shows, including *Today, Good Morning America, The Rachael Ray Show, The Biggest Loser, Nightline*, and many others. As one of the first dietitians to become board certified as a specialist in sports dietetics (CSSD), she has consulted for several professional sports teams, including the Yankees, Rangers, Rays, and Phillies. Cynthia also writes as a freelancer, columnist, and recipe developer for numerous media outlets and, since 2013, has served as contributing nutrition editor at *HEALTH* magazine—a role she has also held at *Shape* magazine and similarly as nutrition director at *Prevention* magazine. Finally, she maintains a private practice in both Manhattan and Los Angeles for counseling individual clients.

Education and Training

Cynthia has a bachelor's degree in nutrition/dietetics and a master's degree in nutrition science with a concentration in community counseling, both from Syracuse University. She also earned a master's degree in public health with a concentration in community and family health education at the University of South Florida. As a long-standing media resource, Cynthia's prior experiences are extensive and span every aspect of communication. She has also worked in medical centers, universities, and fitness/wellness centers in New York, California, Florida, and Texas.

Giving Back to the Profession

Cynthia recalls, "I was recently at a dietetics meeting and was introduced to a new colleague as a nontraditional dietitian. It made me smile but also made me think, 'Is the definition of nontraditional becoming traditional?' I know many dietitians who are involved in unique projects, far outside the walls of a hospital or long-term-care facility. In this field, we can be as inventive as we want to be, and there is enough work to go around for all of us. If you have a passion for this field, you will love what you do, and do it well. As a result, you'll enjoy shaping the profession, and many opportunities will come your way."

In this light, Cynthia's role in shaping the profession includes six years of service as a national media spokesperson for the Academy. While living in Tampa, FL, she was active in the Tampa Dietetic Association, for which she served as president, webmaster, and media rep, as well as corresponding secretary. Cynthia is a member of several DPGs, including SCAN, Vegetarian Nutrition (VN), Dietitians in Integrative and Functional Medicine (DIFM), and Hunger and Environmental Nutrition (HEN). With her passion for sports nutrition, Cynthia is also an active member of the American College of Sports Medicine.

Cynthia Sass's Words of Wisdom

Nutrition is one of the most dynamic and diverse fields because food and nutrition are linked to nearly every aspect of life, at every age. That means there are unlimited opportunities to pursue—if you are creative and entrepreneurial.

Never doubt your knowledge and skills—a registered dietitian is the premier food and nutrition expert!

Clinical and Food: Veronica McLymont, PhD, RDN, CDN

Claim to Fame

Veronica McLymont is an accomplished clinical dietitian, well known for her early advocacy of the Academy's Nutrition Care Process, as well as for her work developing evidence-based clinical nutrition practice guidelines and integrated nutrition screening into initial assessment tools. She is the director of food and nutrition services at Memorial Sloan-Kettering Cancer Center in New York, NY. In this role, she developed and implemented a strategic plan to ensure efficient, cost-effective, high-quality services. Her responsibilities include directing operations within the allocated budget, managing the performance of the team and staff, and implementing quality standards and improvement initiatives to meet safety and regulatory requirements. Her past experience includes time as the assistant director of food services at St. Barnabas Hospital in the Bronx, and as the manager of clinical nutrition and patient services, and the director of food and nutrition services at Memorial Sloan-Kettering Cancer Center in New York.

She has received numerous awards, including the following recent honors:

- Isabelle A. Hallahan Award for Excellence in Foodservice Management from the New York State Academy of Nutrition and Dietetics (2013)
- Excellence in Practice—Management Practice Award Academy of Nutrition and Dietetics (2015)

Education and Training

Veronica holds a bachelor of arts in foods and nutrition from Brooklyn College and a master of science in nutrition from Hunter College. She also completed a doctorate in organizational leadership from the University of Maryland Eastern Shore.

Giving Back to the Profession

Veronica observes, "In my first job as a clinical dietitian, I worked diligently and exceeded expectations. My boss noticed and reassigned me to the outpatient clinic, where I worked independently. Networking with the physicians and nurses in the clinic established me as the nutrition expert. Just about every position I've held since then has been due in part to a professional connection. As leaders, dietetics professionals can go very far. Along the way, we must help those who follow to aspire and achieve heights that help meet their own personal mission as well as those of the profession and our organizations."

Veronica's contributions to the food and nutrition profession have included the following:

- Nominating Committee chair, New York State Dietetic Association
- President, Westchester/Rockland Dietetic Association
- Chair, Nominating Committee for the Clinical Nutrition Management DPG
- Director-at-large, Clinical Nutrition Management DPG
- President, New Chapter for the Association of Healthcare Professionals (AHF-NY)
- Author, nutrition chapter for textbook *Cancer Rehabilitation: Principles and Practice* (2009)

Veronica McLymont's Words of Wisdom

Be resilient, and adapt to change for your personal and professional goals.

The field of dietetics is dynamic and evolving at a rapid pace. Organizations are looking for top performers to join their teams. One way to jump-start your personal and professional growth and take greater responsibility for your career is to expand your networks and build relationships.

Dietetics Leadership / Strategic Planning: Marianne Smith Edge, MS, RD, FADA

Claim to Fame

Marianne Smith Edge is senior advisor, science and consumer insights, for the International Food Information Council (IFIC) in Washington, DC, a nonprofit organization that communicates science-based information on nutrition and food safety. From 2010 to 2015, she served as senior vice president, nutrition and food safety. In this role, Marianne directed the overall nutrition and food safety strategic initiatives of the organization and served as spokesperson on various nutrition, food safety, and health issues. Prior to this, Marianne was owner and president of MSE & Associates, LLC, a nutrition communication and strategic planning consulting firm. Her expertise spans consumer health and wellness research, policy issues, food allergies, nutrition and aging, and strategic positioning of nutritional products and services. Marianne is a group facilitator, developer of workshops and seminars, author, and nationally and internationally recognized speaker. Her 25 years of experience have led to many honors, notably including the Academy of Nutrition and Dietetics 2009 Medallion Award.

Education and Training

Marianne holds a bachelor's of science in dietetics from the University of Kentucky and a master's degree in public health–nutrition from Western Kentucky University. In August 2009, she earned a certification in appreciative inquiry from the Weatherhead School of Management, Case Western Reserve University. In her career, she has served on the US Deparmtent of Agriculture National Research, Extension, Education, and Economics Advisory Board; been a member of the University of Kentucky Board of Trustees; and worked as producer of a family and consumer science television program for the University of Kentucky College of Agriculture Extension Service.

Giving Back to the Profession

Marianne is a past president of the Academy, among numerous other leadership positions within the Academy DPGs, the House of Delegates, and the Ethics Committee, as well as other collaborative task forces. Other professional memberships include the Institute for Food Technologists (IFT), American Society for Nutrition, and the Obesity Society. The following career reflections explain her inspiration and dedication to the profession.

"Since entering the dietetics field 34 years ago, I have learned that establishing a viable business requires networking, staying on the cutting edge of your area of expertise, and understanding that dietetics is a business. Throughout my career, connecting with colleagues has led to career advancement, professional collaborations, and acquisition of a wealth of additional knowledge.

"In particular, my involvement with Dietetics in Health Care Communities DPG was the springboard to my long-standing commitment to the profession and the Academy of Nutrition and Dietetics. Professional growth opportunities, from dietetics practice groups to the House of Delegates and other association-wide committees, provided the foundation for my service with the Academy of Nutrition and Dietetics Board of Directors, as House of Delegates speaker, and as Academy president. Each of these roles has provided me with valuable experience with strategic planning, knowledge-based strategic governance, association management, board facilitation, and member development. The knowledge and leadership skills I have gained are priceless!"

Marianne Smith Edge's Words of Wisdom

Leadership is about giving of yourself to make an organization, profession, or your personal life better for all. It's about doing the right thing.

Dietetics Leadership/Nutrition Informatics: Marty Yadrick, MBI, MS, RDN, FAND

Claim to Fame

Marty Yadrick is director of nutrition informatics for Computrition, Inc, based in West Hills, CA, a company that specializes in foodservice and nutrition care management software solutions. Marty's expertise is in the emerging practice area of nutrition informatics—described as "the intersection of information, nutrition, and technology." In his role at Computrition, Marty assists the business development team as content expert on the nutrition care management functions of the software. This involves participating in software demonstrations, both on-site and via the Web; assisting with requests for proposals; and navigating emerging trends in technology that impact the food and nutrition departments of hospitals, long-term-care facilities, and other types of foodservice operations.

Education and Training

Marty received his bachelor of science at Colorado State University and completed his dietetic internship and master of science in dietetics at the University of Kansas Medical Center. He has also earned a master's degree in business administration from the University of Missouri–Kansas City and, most recently, a master of biomedical informatics from Oregon Health & Science University.

Giving Back to the Profession

Marty remembers, "I always had an interest in the role of nutrition in wellness and prevention of chronic disease. My older sister is a dietitian, and she increased my awareness of nutrition as a career option." Now, 35 years after he began pursuing his own career in nutrition and dietetics, Marty has accumulated an impressive history of volunteer leadership roles. Most notably, Marty is a past president of the Academy (2008–2009).

In recent years, Marty has devoted his time to being a co-instructor for the nutrition-focused 10 x 10 introductory course in biomedical informatics offered annually by the Academy in conjunction with Oregon Health & Science University and the American Medical Informatics Association. He is also a member of the Academy of Nutrition and Dietetics Health Informatics Infrastructure Advisory Workgroup and the Nutrition Fast Healthcare Interoperability Resources Project.

Marty Yadrick's Words of Wisdom

It's so important that our profession stay science based and that we practice based on evidence. Don't let social media sway you away from the source. It's easy to be influenced by what's popular in the media, but science always rules.

Agriculture & Food Systems: Jennie Schmidt, MS, RD

Claim to Fame

Jennie Schmidt is a dietitian, farmer, certified pesticide applicator, and a self-proclaimed "Ag-vocate"—an advocate for agriculture. While attending graduate school and raising a family, Jennie was drawn into working on her family's farm between semesters when the kids were at school, as sometimes the farm was short-handed and she was needed to drive a piece of equipment. Soon it became a passion, and Jennie transitioned into the family business full-time. She connected her training as a dietitian to the direct production of food from the land. When asked why she "threw away all those years of training as a dietitian," Jennie responds: "I practice 'applied nutrition' every day by growing your food. I still am a registered dietitian literally practicing in the (dirt) field of food production." Thus, her designation as a "Foodie Farmer" was born. Jennie eats, lives, and breathes food production on 2,000 highly diversified acres on the eastern shore of Maryland where her family grows corn, soybeans, wheat, barley, hay, tomatoes, green beans, and wine grapes. Visit her blog, The Foodie Farmer, at http://thefoodiefarmer.blogspot.com.

Education and Training

Jennie graduated from the University of Massachusetts, Amherst, with a bachelor's degree in human nutrition and food science and a certification in international agriculture. At this point in her life, Jennie had no intentions of being a dietitian. She had worked tobacco fields in western Massachusetts as a young teen, had helped on a dairy farm, and was a dedicated 4H member, but she had always felt a pull toward agriculture. Instead of doing a dietetic internship,

Jennie moved to Botswana, Africa, under a 2 year contract with the US Department of Agriculture 4H Youth Development Project, helping to develop a 4H-equivalent program. In addition to working with school–based 4H gardening projects to grow food for the school meal program—and because of her degree in nutrition—Jennie was assigned to work in the village health clinics conducting pediatric health and nutrition assessments. Once her contract ended, Jennie decided a degree in nutrition wasn't particularly useful without the dietetian credentials. She completed her internship at UMASS Memorial Medical Center, in Worcester, MA, and immediately took a clinical job at a hospital on the eastern shore of Maryland, drawn there by her now husband. After 10 years in clinical practice, Jennie enrolled in graduate school at the University of Delaware to focus on a degree in food and agriculture biotechnology. With this degree, Jennie works as a nutrient management consultant, writing manure and fertilizer plans for farmers, and a certified pesticide applicator. Jennie delved into the agronomics of crop production and plant biology and found that the systems were woven in a way similar to the relationship between nutrition and the human biological system. Jennie credits her strong foundation in science as a dietitian as essential in helping her become a good farmer.

Giving Back to the Profession

Jennie has focused years of her work on the intersection of food, agriculture, nutrition, and health. She is a long-standing member of the HEN DPG and has served on the Academy of Nutrition and Dietetics Advanced Technology in Food Production Evidence Analysis Library workgroup, as Past-President of the Eastern Shore Chapter of the Maryland Academy of Nutrition and Dietetics, and most recently on the Academy of Nutrition and Dietetics Future of Food Initiative. She is also an Academy Dietitian Farmer and has delivered numerous presentations on food and agriculture to help the profession embrace its food roots.

Jennie's professional food and nutrition contributions include the following:

- President and first female board member of the Maryland Grain Producers Utilization Board
- Farm Mom of the Year
- Maryland Outstanding Young Dietitian of the Year
- Maryland Governor's Agriculture Hall of Fame
- Maryland Wine Association Outstanding Grower of the Year

Jennie Schmidt's Words of Wisdom

Farmers are like dietitians to crops or livestock. Farmers are the front end of nutrition as it is grown in the field, while dietitians are on the back end of nutrition as it relates to consumption. Farmers and dietitians are professionals along the same food continuum.

Farmers comprise only 1% of the US population. Thus fewer and fewer people can relate to how their food gets from the field to their fork.

I want my farm as safe as you want it because I actually live there.

A Special Partnership: Tammy Lakatos Shames, RD, and Elysse ("Lyssie") Lakatos, RD—The Nutrition Twins

Claim to Fame

Tammy Lakatos Shames and Elysse ("Lyssie") Lakatos are RDs, certified personal trainers, and the twin sister co-owners of an innovative nutrition company, The Nutrition Twins. In addition to their identical features, they also share a passion for helping people improve their health through lifestyle-focused behavior modification—a passion that morphed into an endeavor to affect millions of people.

Now, with 15 years of experience, Tammy and Lyssie take a unique approach to nutrition counseling, corporate lecturing, writing, media appearances, and consulting for multinational food companies. They have worked with more than 200 corporations and with thousands of clients. Drawing from their experiences, the sisters have coauthored multiple diet and nutrition advice books, most recently *The Nutrition Twins' Veggie Cure: Expert Advice and Tantalizing Recipes for Health, Energy and Beauty* (2014). In radio and TV, they have been featured regularly as nutrition experts on the Discovery Health channel, Fox News channel, NBC, Bravo, WABC-TV, WPIX-TV, CBS, The Learning Channel, FitTV, Oxygen Network, Life and Style, Court TV, *Fox & Friends*, and *Good Day New York*. They are writers for Livestrong. com and the American Council on Exercise (ACE) and are sought-after contributors to a range of print and digital publications, from magazines to online resources for WebMD, MSN, WeightWatchers, and more.

Education and Training

Tammy and Lyssie are graduates of the University of Maryland and completed their dietetic internships at Emory University and Meredith College. They are also ACE-certified personal trainers.

Giving Back to the Profession

To give back to the profession, the twins are members of the Academy and the New York State Academy affiliate. They are also active in the following DPGs: SCAN; DIFM; and Nutrition Entrepreneurs. The twins have appeared as speakers for professional organizations, for example, as the keynote for the New Jersey Academy of Nutrition and Dietetics annual meeting and as the featured presenters at the International Society of Sports Nutrition's annual conference.

The Nutrition Twins' Words of Wisdom

Follow your passion. You won't have any regrets. Pursue what excites you, and put everything you have into achieving your dreams.

Q & A with the Nutrition Twins

Kyle and Milton: Apart from your twin status, what makes you different from your competition?

Tammy: Good question. We don't really see our colleagues as competition. We are thankful to be surrounded by great dietitians—we can all learn from each other. Successful RDNs inspire us to work harder. I think the biggest thing that separates us is that we do not limit ourselves to just counseling or writing; we love to do it all, so we do. We also personalize everything we do and use our own style of counseling/lecturing, etc, which differentiates us from others.

K & M: Did you both decide at the same time that you wanted to become dietitians?

Lyssie: I always say I decided first, and since I am 17 minutes older, Tammy wanted to do whatever I did. However, we were both always intrigued by food and its link to health because we were always athletic. I think we both decided around our first year of college, when we were getting a little taste of college life and trying to survive on dining hall food.

K & M: How has your nutrition education helped you as entrepreneurs?

Tammy: It has given me a solid foundation, which has given me the confidence to be an entrepreneur.

Lyssie: While experiencing clinical, foodservice management, and community rotations during my internship and seeing all of the different avenues that one could take as a dietitian, I learned that there were several things I enjoyed doing and that I wanted my practice to incorporate each of those aspects. Having the confidence in my ability as a nutritionist gave me the courage to set out as an entrepreneur.

K & M: Who helped you the most during your career?

Tammy: Actually, Lyssie has helped me more than anyone else. After all, she is my partner in crime. I did have a lot of other mentors, especially when I was in school, including my professors and my internship director, Debbie Clegg.

Lyssie: There have been many helpful people in my career, but one of the most instrumental was Ansley Hudson, a dietitian I shadowed during my internship. She worked in private practice as a consultant for professional athletes and managed corporate wellness initiatives. She was a very hard worker, and I quickly realized that you have to be motivated and disciplined in order to succeed as an entrepreneur. I began my career by structuring it somewhat like hers. I also remember how much she helped me, and I try to help other interns or people in the profession as much as she did for me.

K & M: Tell us about your successful private practice.

Tammy: I view success as happiness and being excited about waking up every morning and going to work. We love what we do. No two days are ever the same. The variety excites us.

Lyssie: Our practice is actually somewhat like Ansley's was, since we modeled it after hers. We have a variety of clients who see us individually. We provide larger seminars for corporations in New York City, some of which are 6-, 8-, and 10-week nutrition programs. We also do media and TV appearances as nutrition experts. And nowadays, we spend a lot of time trying to motivate and empower our followers on social media and through our writing.

K & M: What motivates you?

Tammy: I am motivated by people who want to improve their lives and want to become healthier. It excites me to help them make their lives happier.

Lyssie: I like the way it feels to help people, and this motivates me. Other dietitians also motivate me. I am also motivated by success, which for me is feeling as though I am continually growing and improving.

K & M: You both have been featured regularly as the nutrition experts for many prominent media outlets. You both must have a media agent. What's the most important piece of advice you can give to anyone who wants to work with the media?

Tammy: It actually wasn't an agent who lined us up with these opportunities. It's all about networking and hard work and persistence. Do not get discouraged. One day a door will open for you, and then many will follow. Even though an agent isn't always nec-essary, we do have an agent, they're really helpful when it comes to negotiating contracts.

Lyssie: I agree with Tammy. Do not give up. If you pitch an idea but you don't hear back, it doesn't necessarily mean that they aren't in-terested; it just means they are busy. Even if they aren't interested, pitch a different idea!

K & M: Do you plan to attend graduate school? Why or why not?

Tammy: I would love to. I know it sounds cliché, but knowledge is power. Our field changes so much day to day with new research, and it really is important to stay on top of it. The only thing holding me back is finding the time in a crazy work schedule.

Lyssie: Absolutely! I love learning and feel like I still want to learn so much more. Currently we are taking business classes.

K & M: What do you both want to be doing in 10 years?

Tammy: I love what I do now, and if I am still doing it in 10 years, I would be thrilled!

Lyssie: This career has been an amazing whirlwind, and as I am faced with so many different amazing opportunities, I would be thrilled if any pan out and each could take me into an entirely dif-ferent future.

Afterword

HI THERE! IT'S US, KYLE AND MILTON AGAIN. IF YOU'RE reading this, we hope it's because you've recently earned your RDN credential and have kept this guide by your side along the way.

As we said at the start, we wish we'd had something like this book when we were learning the ropes. We hope we've made it easier for you to navigate your way to the RDN credential and that you're now ready and energized to make the most of your career! Being an RDN is a rewarding career choice, and we hope you love it as much as we do.

If you've taken our advice, you are probably already volunteering for our profession (or working on it), and putting your networking skills to good use, which means we'll run into each other soon enough. Though we are nearly 67,000 strong (in the United States alone), the nutrition and dietetics community is relatively small (in a good way), so it's likely our paths will cross someday. When you see us, please say hello!

We genuinely hope this guide has been a valuable companion to you. Good luck, and thank you for all the work you'll be doing in the name of nutrition.

Our best wishes,
—Kyle and Milton

Leading Nutrition-Related Organizations

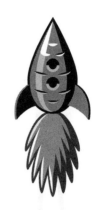

Academy of Nutrition and Dietetics
120 South Riverside Plaza,
Suite 2000
Chicago, IL 60606-6995
Phone: 800/877-1600
www.eatright.org

American Association of Diabetes Educators
200 W. Madison Street, Suite 800
Chicago, IL 60606
Phone: 800/338-3633
www.diabeteseducator.org

American College of Sports Medicine
401 West Michigan Street
Indianapolis, IN 46202-3233
Phone: 317/637-9200
www.acsm.org

American Diabetes Association
1701 North Beauregard Street
Alexandria, VA 22311
Phone: 800/342-2383
www.diabetes.org

American Heart Association
7272 Greenville Avenue
Dallas, TX 75231
Phone: 800/242-8721
www.heart.org

American Society for Nutrition
9211 Corporate Boulevard,
Suite 300
Rockville, MD 20850
Phone: 240/428-3650
www.nutrition.org

American Society for Parenteral and Enteral Nutrition (A.S.P.E.N.)
8630 Fenton Street, Suite 412
Silver Spring, MD 20910
Phone: 301/587-6315
E-mail: aspen@nutritioncare.org
www.nutritioncare.org

Association of Nutrition and Foodservice Professionals
406 Surrey Woods Drive
St. Charles, IL 60174
Phone: 800/323-1908
www.anfponline.org

Dietitians of Canada
480 University Avenue, Suite 604
Toronto, Ontario, Canada M5G 1V2
Phone: 416/596-0857
E-mail: contactus@dietitians.ca
www.dietitians.ca

Gerontological Society of America
1220 L Street NW, Suite 901
Washington, DC 20005
Phone: 202/842-1275
www.geron.org

Institute of Food Technologists
525 W. Van Buren, Suite 1000
Chicago, IL 60607
Phone: 312/782-8424
www.ift.org

International Association of Culinary Professionals
45 Rockefeller Plaza, Suite 2000
New York, NY 10111
Phone: 866/358-4951
www.iacp.com

National Restaurant Association
2055 L Street NW, Suite 700
Washington, DC 20036
Phone: 800/424-5156
www.restaurant.org

Obesity Society
1110 Bonifant Street, Suite 500
Silver Spring, MD 20910
Phone: 301/563-6526
www.obesity.org

Retail Dietitians Business Alliance
3015 Main Street, Suite 320
Santa Monica, CA 90405
Phone: 310/392-0448
www.retaildietitians.com

School Nutrition Association
120 Waterfront Street, Suite 300
National Harbor, MD 20745
Phone: 301/686-3100
E-mail: servicecenter@school
nutrition.org
www.schoolnutrition.org

Society for Nutrition Education and Behavior
9100 Purdue Road, Suite 200
Indianapolis, IN 46268
Phone: 317/328-4627
www.sneb.org

Index

volunteering, 17, 31, 105–106

Web sites,
> for annual conferences, 83
> on certification programs, 93
> for financial aid, 66–67
> for job search, 99
> for nutrition organizations, 10, 89
> on professional development, 84
> for publications, 91
> on RDN exam, 71
> for salary negotiation, 105
> on telehealth, 9

weight management, specialization in, 3
Winkler, Marion F., 119–121
work samples, for job application, 103
Writer's Market, 110
writing for publication, 108–111
writing samples, for internship application, 42

Yadrick, Marty, 145–147

Zelman, Kathleen M., 116–117